Acute Ischemic Stroke

Guest Editors

LAUREN M. NENTWICH, MD
BRENDAN G. MAGAURAN Jr, MD, MBA
JOSEPH H. KAHN, MD, FACEP

EMERGENCY MEDICINE CLINICS OF NORTH AMERICA

www.emed.theclinics.com

Consulting Editor
AMAL MATTU, MD

August 2012 • Volume 30 • Number 3

SAUNDERS an imprint of ELSEVIER, Inc.

W.B. SAUNDERS COMPANY

A Division of Elsevier Inc.

1600 John F. Kennedy Boulevard ● Suite 1800 ● Philadelphia, Pennsylvania 19103-2899

http://www.theclinics.com

EMERGENCY MEDICINE CLINICS OF NORTH AMERICA Volume 30, Number 3
August 2012 ISSN 0733-8627, ISBN-13: 978-1-4557-4939-3

Editor: Patrick Manley
Developmental Editor: Donald Mumford

Emergency Medicine Clinics of North America (ISSN 0733-8627) is published quarterly by Elsevier Inc., 360 Park Avenue South, New York, NY, 10010-1710. Months of issue are February, May, August, and November. Business and Editorial Offices: 1600 John F. Kennedy Boulevard, Suite 1800, Philadelphia, PA 19103-2899. Customer Service Office: 6277 Sea Harbor Drive, Orlando, FL 32887-4800. Periodicals postage paid at New York, NY, and additional mailing offices. Subscription prices are $142.00 per year (US students), $281.00 per year (US individuals), $478.00 per year (US institutions), $201.00 per year (international students), $404.00 per year (international individuals), $576.00 per year (international institutions), $201.00 per year (Canadian students), $347.00 per year (Canadian individuals), and $576.00 per year (Canadian institutions). International air speed delivery is included in all *Clinics'* subscription prices. All prices are subject to change without notice. **POSTMASTER:** Send address changes to *Emergency Medicine Clinics of North America*, Elsevier Periodicals Customer Service, 11830 Westline Industrial Drive, St. Louis, MO 63146. Customer Service (orders, claims, online, change of address): Elsevier Periodicals Customer Service, 11830 Westline Industrial Drive, St. Louis, MO 63146. Tel: 1-800-654-2452 (U.S. and Canada); 314-453-7041 (outside U.S. and Canada). Fax: 314-453-5170. E-mail: journalscustomerservice-usa@elsevier.com (for print support); journalsonline support-usa@elsevier.com (for online support).

Reprints. For copies of 100 or more of articles in this publication, please contact the Commercial Reprints Department, Elsevier Inc., 360 Park Avenue South, New York, NY 10010-1710. Tel.: 212-633-3812; Fax: 212-462-1935; E-mail: reprints@elsevier.com.

Emergency Medicine Clinics of North America is covered in *MEDLINE/PubMed (Index Medicus), Current Contents/Clinical Medicine, EMBASE/Excerpta Medica, BIOSIS, SciSearch, CINAHL, ISI/BIOMED,* and *Research Alert.*

Printed and bound by CPI Group (UK) Ltd, Croydon, CR0 4YY

Transferred to Digital Print 2012

Contributors

CONSULTING EDITOR

AMAL MATTU, MD, FAAEM, FACEP
Program Director, Emergency Medicine Residency; Professor, Department of Emergency
Medicine, University of Maryland School of Medicine, Baltimore, Maryland

GUEST EDITORS

LAUREN M. NENTWICH, MD
Attending Physician, Department of Emergency Medicine, Boston Medical Center;
Instructor of Emergency Medicine, Boston University School of Medicine, Boston,
Massachusetts

BRENDAN G. MAGAURAN Jr, MD, MBA
Department of Emergency Medicine, Boston Medical Center; Assistant Professor of
Emergency Medicine, Boston University School of Medicine, Boston, Massachusetts

JOSEPH H. KAHN, MD, FACEP
Director, Medical Student Education, Department of Emergency Medicine, Boston
Medical Center; Associate Professor of Emergency Medicine, Boston University School
of Medicine, Boston, Massachusetts

AUTHORS

JOSEPH D. BURNS, MD
Assistant Professor of Neurology and Neurosurgery, Departments of Neurology and
Neurosurgery, Boston Medical Center, Boston University School of Medicine, Boston,
Massachusetts

J. ALFREDO CACERES, MD
Department of Neurology, Massachusetts General Hospital, Boston, Massachusetts

ANNA M. CERVANTES-ARSLANIAN, MD
Department of Neurology, Boston University School of Medicine/Boston Medical Center,
Boston, Massachusetts

CHRISTINA DEFUSCO, ANP
Department of Neurology, Boston Medical Center, Boston University School of Medicine,
Boston, Massachusetts

DAVID H. DORFMAN, MD
Division of Pediatric Emergency Medicine, Boston University School of Medicine/Boston
Medical Center, Boston, Massachusetts

JONATHAN A. EDLOW, MD, FACEP
Department of Emergency Medicine, Beth Israel Deaconess Medical Center, Professor of Medicine, Harvard Medical School, Boston, Massachusetts

CHARISE L. FREUNDLICH, MD
Division of Pediatric Emergency Medicine, Boston University School of Medicine/Boston Medical Center, Boston, Massachusetts

JOSHUA N. GOLDSTEIN, MD, PhD
Assistant Professor, Harvard Medical School; Department of Emergency Medicine, Massachusetts General Hospital, Boston, Massachusetts

DEBORAH M. GREEN, MD
Clinical Associate Professor of Neurology and Neurosurgery, Departments of Neurology and Neurosurgery, Boston Medical Center, Boston University School of Medicine, Boston, Massachusetts

JOSEPH H. KAHN, MD, FACEP
Director, Medical Student Education, Department of Emergency Medicine, Boston Medical Center; Associate Professor of Emergency Medicine, Boston University School of Medicine, Boston, Massachusetts

RICKY KUE, MD, MPH, FACEP
Associate Medical Director, Boston Emergency Medical Services, Office of Research, Training and Quality Improvement; Assistant Professor of Emergency Medicine, Boston University School of Medicine, Boston, Massachusetts

BRENDAN G. MAGAURAN Jr, MD, MBA
Department of Emergency Medicine, Boston Medical Center; Assistant Professor of Emergency Medicine, Boston University School of Medicine, Boston, Massachusetts

KERRY K. MCCABE, MD
Assistant Professor, Department of Emergency Medicine, Boston Medical Center, Boston University School of Medicine, Boston, Massachusetts

LAUREN M. NENTWICH, MD
Attending Physician, Department of Emergency Medicine, Boston Medical Center; Assistant Professor of Emergency Medicine, Boston University School of Medicine, Boston, Massachusetts

KRISTEN METIVIER, MD
Department of Neurology, Boston Medical Center, Boston University School of Medicine, Boston, Massachusetts

THANH NGOC NGUYEN, MD, FRCPc
Director, Interventional Neuroradiology; Assistant Professor, Departments of Neurology, Neurosurgery, and Radiology, Boston Medical Center, Boston University School of Medicine, Boston, Massachusetts

MEAGHAN NITKA, MD
Senior Resident, Department of Emergency Medicine, Boston Medical Center, Boston University School of Medicine, Boston, Massachusetts

JONATHAN S. OLSHAKER, MD, FACEP, FAAEM
Professor and Chair, Chief, Department of Emergency Medicine, Boston Medical Center, Boston University School of Medicine, Boston, Massachusetts

JOSEPH R. PARE, MD
Department of Emergency Medicine, Boston Medical Center, Boston, Massachusetts

JILLIAN M. PERRY, MD
Senior Resident, Department of Emergency Medicine, Boston Medical Center, Boston, Massachusetts

JEFFREY I. SCHNEIDER, MD, FACEP
Assistant Professor of Emergency Medicine, Residency Program Director, Department of Emergency Medicine, Boston Medical Center, Boston University School of Medicine, Boston, Massachusetts

MATTHEW S. SIKET, MD, MS
Department of Emergency Medicine, Instructor of Surgery, Harvard Medical School, Massachusetts General Hospital, Boston, Massachusetts

JASMEET SINGH, MD, MPHA
Department of Neurology, Boston Medical Center, Boston University School of Medicine, Boston, Massachusetts

ALAINA STECK, MD, FACEP
Department of Emergency Medicine, Boston University School of Medicine, Boston, Massachusetts

WILLIAM VELOZ, MD
Resident Physician, Department of Emergency Medicine, Boston University Medical Center, Boston, Massachusetts

JOSEPH R. PANE, MD
Department of Emergency Medicine, Boston Medical Center, Boston, Massachusetts

JILLIAN M. PERRY, MD
Senior Resident, Department of Emergency Medicine, Boston Medical Center, Boston, Massachusetts

JEFFREY I. SCHNEIDER, MD, FACEP
Assistant Professor of Emergency Medicine, Residency Program Director, Department of Emergency Medicine, Boston Medical Center, Boston University School of Medicine, Boston, Massachusetts

MATTHEW S. SIKET, MD, MS
Department of Emergency Medicine, Instructor of Surgery, Harvard Medical School, Massachusetts General Hospital, Boston, Massachusetts

JASMEET SINGH, MD, MPHA
Department of Neurology, Boston Medical Center, Boston University School of Medicine, Boston, Massachusetts

ALAINA STECK, MD, FACEP
Department of Emergency Medicine, Boston University School of Medicine, Boston, Massachusetts

WILLIAM VILOZ, MD
Resident Physician, Department of Emergency Medicine, Boston University Medical Center, Boston, Massachusetts

Contents

> Stroke should not solely be considered a disease of the elderly, and racial disparities are most evident among young adults. Acute stroke can present at any age and it is important to be familiar with the evaluation and treatment of stroke to provide timely care. The National Institute of Health Stroke Scale helps physicians objectively evaluate stroke patients. This article presents an overview of basic information on neuroanatomy, pathophysiology, and stroke syndromes.

> Significant advances in the early management of ischemic stroke have been made since the 1995 National Institute of Neurologic Disorders and Stroke data demonstrated the benefit of early intravenous administration of tissue plasminogen activator to select patients with acute ischemic stroke within a 3-hour onset window of suspected stroke symptoms. One concept in stroke care that has become better understood is the importance of time management and the ability to deliver patients with acute stroke to appropriate care as soon as possible. Minimizing delay to definitive therapy remains the current focus in the prehospital phase of stroke care.

> This article addresses the recognition and management of acute ischemic stroke. It includes a discussion of cerebrovascular anatomy, common ischemic stroke syndromes, and central venous thrombosis. Extensive attention is paid to the initial emergency department management of stroke, addressing medical and systems issues, and treatment of ischemic stroke by thrombolysis.

> This article reviews the various imaging modalities available for the evaluation of patients presenting with a potential stroke syndrome, specifically

acute ischemic stroke, intracerebral hemorrhage, and subarachnoid hemorrhage. It reviews the various computed tomography (CT) modalities, including noncontrast brain CT (NCCT), CT angiography, and CT perfusion. It discusses multimodal magnetic resonance imaging in the evaluation of patients with acute stroke, including diffusion-weighted imaging, T2-weighted sequences/fluid-attenuated inversion recovery, magnetic resonance angiography, perfusion-weighted imaging, and gradient-recalled echo. At the end of this article, a brief review on how to read an NCCT geared toward the emergency physician is included.

Jeffrey I. Schneider and Jonathan S. Olshaker

Dizzy patients present a significant diagnostic challenge to the emergency clinician. The discrimination between peripheral and central causes is important and will inform subsequent diagnostic evaluation and treatment. Isolated vertigo can be the only initial symptom of a posterior circulation stroke. The sensation of imbalance especially raises this possibility. Research involving strokes of the posterior circulation has lagged behind that of the anterior cerebral circulation. Investigations of the last 20 years, using new technologies in brain imaging in combination with detailed clinical studies, have revolutionized our understanding of the clinical presentation, causes, treatments, and prognosis of posterior circulation ischemia.

Jasmeet Singh and Thanh Ngoc Nguyen

Acute ischemic stroke is recognized as the third leading cause of death in the United States; improved treatments for management are important to reduce disability and death. The standard of care of acute stroke therapy has been reperfusion/recanalization of the occluded vessels using pharmacologic management, endovascular management, or a combination approach. Significant improvements have been made in the management with the use of endovascular therapy. This article reviews the literature on the endovascular and neurosurgical management of patients presenting with acute ischemic stroke and presents current evidence-based guidelines for endovascular or neurosurgical interventions outlined for management of ischemic stroke.

Joseph D. Burns, Deborah M. Green, Kristen Metivier, and Christina DeFusco

Despite the success of acute reperfusion therapies for the treatment of acute ischemic stroke, only a minority of patients receive such treatment. Even patients who receive reperfusion therapy remain at risk for further neuronal death through progressive infarction and secondary injury mechanisms. The goal of neurocritical care for the patient with acute ischemic stroke is to optimize long-term outcomes by minimizing the amount of brain tissue that is lost to these processes. This is accomplished by optimizing brain perfusion, limiting secondary brain injury, and compensating for associated dysfunction in other organ systems. Because of the rapid and irreversible nature of ischemic brain injury, it is crucial for best neuro-critical care practices to begin as early as possible. Therefore, this chapter will discuss optimal, pragmatic neurocritical care management of patients with acute ischemic stroke during the "golden" emergency department hours from the perspective of the neurointensivist. Major topics include cerebral perfusion optimization; management of cerebral edema; post-thrombolytic care; acute anticoagulation; treatment of commonly associated cardiac and pulmonary complications; fluid, electrolyte and glucose management; the role of induced normothermia and therapeutic hypother-mia; and prophylaxis against common complications.

GOAL STATEMENT
The goal of *Emergency Medicine Clinics of North America* is to keep practicing physicians up to date with current clinical practice in emergency medicine by providing timely articles reviewing the state of the art in patient care.

ACCREDITATION
The *Emergency Medical Clinics of North America* is planned and implemented in accordance with the Essential Areas and Policies of the Accreditation Council for Continuing Medical Education (ACCME) through the joint sponsorship of the University of Virginia School of Medicine and Elsevier. The University of Virginia School of Medicine is accredited by the ACCME to provide continuing medical education for physicians.

The University of Virginia School of Medicine designates this enduring material activity for a maximum of 15 *AMA PRA Category 1 Credit(s)™* for each issue, 60 credits per year. Physicians should claim only the credit commensurate with the extent of their participation in the activity.

The American Medical Association has determined that physicians not licensed in the US who participate in this CME enduring material activity are eligible for a maximum of 15 *AMA PRA Category 1 Credit(s)™* for each issue, 60 credits per year.

The Emergency Medicine Clinics of North America CME program is approved by the American College of Emergency Physicians for 60 hours of ACEP Category I Credit per year.

Credit can be earned by reading the text material, taking the CME examination online at http://www.theclinics.com/home/cme, and completing the evaluation. After taking the test, you will be required to review any and all incorrect answers. Following completion of the test and evaluation, your credit will be awarded and you may print your certificate.

FACULTY DISCLOSURE/CONFLICT OF INTEREST
The University of Virginia School of Medicine, as an ACCME accredited provider, endorses and strives to comply with the Accreditation Council for Continuing Medical Education (ACCME) Standards of Commercial Support, Commonwealth of Virginia statutes, University of Virginia policies and procedures, and associated federal and private regulations and guidelines on the need for disclosure and monitoring of proprietary and financial interests that may affect the scientific integrity and balance of content delivered in continuing medical education activities under our auspices.

The University of Virginia School of Medicine requires that all CME activities accredited through this institution be developed independently and be scientifically rigorous, balanced and objective in the presentation/discussion of its content, theories and practices.

All authors/editors participating in an accredited CME activity are expected to disclose to the readers relevant financial relationships with commercial entities occurring within the past 12 months (such as grants or research support, employee, consultant, stock holder, member of speakers bureau, etc.). The University of Virginia School of Medicine will employ appropriate mechanisms to resolve potential conflicts of interest to maintain the standards of fair and balanced education to the reader. Questions about specific strategies can be directed to the Office of Continuing Medical Education, University of Virginia School of Medicine, Charlottesville, Virginia.

The faculty and staff of the University of Virginia Office of Continuing Medical Education have no financial affiliations to disclose.

The authors/editors listed below have identified no professional or financial affiliations for themselves or their spouse/partner:
Joseph D. Burns, MD; J. Alfredo Caceres, MD; Anna M. Cervantes-Arslanian, MD; Christina DeFusco, ANP; David H. Dorfman, MD; Jonathan A. Edlow, MD; Deborah M. Green, MD; Joseph H. Kahn, MD (Guest Editor); Ricky Kue, MD, MPH, FACEP; Brendan G. Magauran Jr, MD, MBA (Guest Editor); Patrick Manley, (Acquisitions Editor); Amal Mattu, MD, FAAEM, FACEP (Consulting Editor); Kerry K. McCabe, MD; Kristen Metivier, MD; Lauren M. Nentwich, MD (Guest Editor); Thanh Ngoc Nguyen, MD, FRCPc; Meaghan Nitka, MD; Jonathan S. Olshaker, MD; Joseph R. Pare, MD; Jillian M. Perry, MD; Jeffrey I. Schneider, MD; Matthew S. Siket, MD, MS; Jasmeet Singh, MD, MPHA; Alaina Steck, MD, FACEP; William Veloz, MD; and William A. Woods, MD (Test Author).

The authors/editors listed below identified the following professional or financial affiliations for themselves or their spouse/partner:
Charise L. Freundlich, MD is employed by and owns stock in Vertex Pharmaceuticals.
Joshua N. Goldstein, MD, PhD receives research funding and is a consultant for CSL Behring.

Disclosure of Discussion of Non-FDA Approved Uses for Pharmaceutical Products and/or Medical Devices.
The University of Virginia School of Medicine, as an ACCME provider, requires that all faculty presenters identify and disclose any off-label uses for pharmaceutical and medical device products. The University of Virginia School of Medicine recommends that each physician fully review all the available data on new products or procedures prior to clinical use.

TO ENROLL
To enroll in the Emergency Medicine Clinics of North America Continuing Medical Education program, call customer service at 1-800-654-2452 or visit us online at www.theclinics.com/home/cme. The CME program is available to subscribers for an additional fee of $190.00.

Foreword

Acute Ischemic Stroke

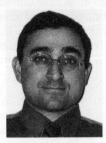

Amal Mattu, MD, FAAEM, FACEP
Consulting Editor

The brain has long been considered the "black box" of the human body. This term reflects the failure of generations of physicians and researchers to understand well the inner workings of the brain. Even as recently as the late 1980s, when I was in medical school, the diagnosis and treatment of "brain conditions" were considered by many of us mostly an exercise in frustration...many diagnoses were educated guesses, and treatment was primarily just supportive therapy and rehabilitation. Stroke was the hallmark disease of the field of neurology, and it typified all of these frustrations: we didn't understand stroke well, we couldn't diagnose it well, and we couldn't treat it well. This frustration existed despite the fact that stroke had long been a leading cause of death in developed countries.

During the past two decades, however, the walls of the black box in which stroke exists have been becoming more transparent. Marked advances in diagnostic imaging have helped us gain a far greater understanding of the different types of stroke and associated conditions that predict stroke. Then in 1995 with the publication of the first major study demonstrating successful thrombolysis in ischemic stroke,[1] the field of neurology abruptly changed. The "black box" mentality we held regarding the brain was disappearing, and the hallmark disease of stroke almost overnight had become easily diagnosable and often treatable. Following the 1995 publication, there has been an explosion of research and publications demonstrating clinical advances in the diagnosis and treatment of stroke. Ironically, a condition which once was easy to maintain an up-to-date knowledge base has now become one with which we emergency physicians have a tough time staying up to date.

Fortunately for us, Drs Kahn, Magauran, and Nentwich have provided in this issue of *Emergency Medicine Clinics of North America* a cutting-edge review of stroke to help us stay up to date. They've assembled an outstanding team to educate us about the latest diagnostic modalities and therapies, from the prehospital arena to the emergency department to the interventional radiology suite to the operating room. A special article is included to review the neuroanatomy and provide clinical correlation to stroke

Emerg Med Clin N Am 30 (2012) xiii–xiv
http://dx.doi.org/10.1016/j.emc.2012.06.008
emed.theclinics.com

syndromes. Articles are also included to address stroke mimics, transient ischemic attacks, and intracranial hemorrhage. Finally, an article is provided to address the rare but devastating strokes that may occur in the pediatric population.

The Guest Editors and authors are to be commended for their hard work. This issue of *Emergency Medicine Clinics of North America* represents an invaluable addition to the emergency medicine literature, one that should be on the bookshelves of all emergency departments and especially all stroke centers in the country. The contributors have helped to tear down the "black box" of the brain and they've demonstrated nicely how far we've come in the diagnosis and management of a previously frustrating condition.

Amal Mattu, MD, FAAEM, FACEP
Department of Emergency Medicine
University of Maryland School of Medicine
110 S. Paca Street, 6th Floor, Suite 200
Baltimore, MD 21201, USA

E-mail address:
amattu@smail.umaryland.edu

REFERENCE

1. Tissue plasminogen activator for acute ischemic stroke. The National Institute of Neurological Disorders and Stroke rt-PA Stroke Study Group. N Engl J Med 1995;333:1581–7.

Preface

Acute Ischemic Stroke

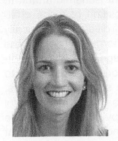 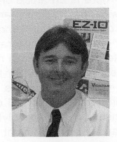 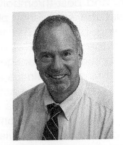

Lauren M. Nentwich, MD   Brendan G. Magauran Jr, MD, MBA   Joseph H. Kahn, MD, FACEP
Guest Editors

Early recognition and aggressive management of acute ischemic stroke (AIS) is an integral part of the practice of Emergency Medicine. Stroke is the fourth leading cause of death, accounting for approximately 134,000 deaths annually, and the leading cause of serious long-term disability in the United States. There are approximately 795,000 strokes annually in the United States and 6.4 million stroke survivors. Many stroke survivors suffer from significant disability with tremendous personal and financial cost to the individual, the family, and the health care system.

The 1995 NINDS rt-PA in acute stroke trial changed the management of AIS from observation and rehabilitation to acute, time-sensitive treatment.[1] Treatment of AIS diagnosed within three hours of symptom onset with thrombolytic therapy offered the first active advance in AIS, and management detailing when and how treatment should be administered in the emergency setting is of paramount importance for the practicing emergency physician.

This edition includes an article on basic neuroanatomy and stroke syndromes, which provides a practical review of neuroanatomy for the practicing physician and outlines common stroke presentations. There is an article reviewing the essential role that prehospital EMS systems play in rapid stroke recognition and treatment. The article on recognition and management of AIS reviews the key steps involved in the rapid evaluation and treatment decisions regarding stroke patients presenting to the emergency department. Since rapid, accurate interpretation of proper neuroimaging is part of the emergency management of stroke patients, we have included an article on neuroimaging that not only reviews available imaging modalities and when to order them, but also includes a step-by-step guide on the interpretation of brain CT by the emergency physician. The article on vertigo, vertebrobasilar disease, and posterior circulation ischemic stroke aids the emergency physician in distinguishing posterior circulation stroke from more benign causes of vertigo. There is also a role for intraarterial thrombolysis, mechanical clot retrieval, and neurosurgery in AIS, and

Emerg Med Clin N Am 30 (2012) xv–xvi
http://dx.doi.org/10.1016/j.emc.2012.06.007
0733-8627/12/$ – see front matter © 2012 Elsevier Inc. All rights reserved.

emed.theclinics.com

these topics are discussed in the article on endovascular and neurosurgical management of stroke. The article on intensive care management of AIS patients addresses some of the difficult management decisions that emergency physicians make when treating patients with AIS, such as blood pressure control, ventilation and oxygenation, and post-thrombolytic care. There is an article on transient ischemic attack to assist the emergency physician with the treatment and disposition of these challenging patients. The treatment of intracranial hemorrhages diverges drastically from the treatment of AIS, and the article on intracranial hemorrhage outlines the recognition and management of life-threatening brain hemorrhage. The article dedicated to stroke mimics alerts the emergency provider to onditions, which appear to be a stroke, but are actually non-vascular conditions such as seizures, migraines, metabolic disturbances and degenerative eurological disorders that require careful diagnostic consideration prior to initiation of thrombolytic therapy. Finally, the article on pediatric stroke reviews the causes and treatment of the increasingly prevalent problem of stroke in the pediatric age group.

In expressing our appreciation for the work associated with this issue, we first and foremost would like to thank all of the authors who made this issue on AIS possible. We would also like to thank Patrick Manley and the staff at Elsevier for their guidance and support. We also thank our families for allowing us the time to assemble and edit this issue. Most of all, we thank those of you who read this issue of *Emergency Medicine Clinics of North America*.

Lauren M. Nentwich, MD

Brendan G. Magauran Jr, MD, MBA

Joseph H. Kahn, MD, FACEP
Department of Emergency Medicine
Boston Medical Center
Boston University School of Medicine
1 Boston Medical Center Place
Boston, MA 02118, USA

E-mail addresses:
lauren.nentwich@bmc.org (L.M. Nentwich)
Brendan.magauran@bmc.org (B.G. Magauran)
jkahn@bu.edu (J.H. Kahn)

Basic Neuroanatomy and Stroke Syndromes

Joseph R. Pare, MD[a], Joseph H. Kahn, MD[b],*

KEYWORDS

- Stroke • Stroke syndromes • Neuroanatomy and stroke
- Pathophysiology and stroke

KEY POINTS

- Middle cerebral artery occlusion in dominant hemisphere causes aphasia and contralateral motor and sensory deficits.
- Vertebrobasilar occlusion may present with dizziness and ataxia, then progress to quadriplegia and coma.
- Carotid artery dissection, a cause of stroke in young people, may present with Horner syndrome.
- Cerebral venous thrombosis may present as headache, seizure, or coma.

INTRODUCTION TO STROKE

Acute stroke care is a cornerstone of emergency medicine practice owing to its significant morbidity and mortality. There are an estimated 795,000 strokes annually and 6.4 million American stroke survivors.[1] Stroke is the third leading cause of death nationally, and accounts for a calculated 134,000 deaths annu\ally.[1]

Of those people affected, it is helpful to be aware of the significant disparities within the field of stroke. Black and Hispanic/Latino Americans have a higher incidence of all types of stroke when compared with Caucasians. Studies report stroke incidence is nearly twice as high for blacks as compared with whites.[2] Additionally, stroke should not solely be considered a disease of the elderly, and again racial disparities are most evident among young adults.[2] Acute stroke can present at any age and it is important to be familiar with the evaluation and treatment of stroke to provide timely care.[3] The National Institute of Health Stroke Scale (NIHSS) helps physicians objectively evaluate stroke patients (**Table 1**). This article presents an overview of basic information on neuroanatomy, pathophysiology, and stroke syndromes.

[a] Department of Emergency Medicine, Boston Medical Center, 1 Boston Medical Center Place, Boston, MA 02118, USA; [b] Medical Student Education, Department of Emergency Medicine, Boston Medical Center, Boston University School of Medicine, 1 Boston Medical Center Place, Boston, MA 02118, USA
* Corresponding author.
E-mail address: jkahn@bu.edu

Emerg Med Clin N Am 30 (2012) 601–615
doi:10.1016/j.emc.2012.05.004
0733-8627/12/$ – see front matter © 2012 Elsevier Inc. All rights reserved.

therefore this lobe is primarily responsible for vision. Any damage to the cerebral cortex may result in clinical presentations with corresponding loss to these anatomic functions.[7]

The basal ganglia primarily coordinate movement and are composed of the caudate, putamen, and globus pallidus. The limbic system is composed of the amygdala, cingulate gyrus, and the hippocampus. The amygdala and cingulate gyrus are important in memory and emotion, whereas the hippocampus is responsible for memory and learning. These structures are located internal to the cerebral cortex and closer to the core of the brain.[7]

Diencephalon

This portion of the brain is the area between the brain stem and the cerebrum. This portion is composed of the thalamus, hypothalamus, and pituitary and pineal glands. The thalamus is critical to sensory function, as almost all sensory information passes through this portion of the brain before being directed to the cerebrum. The thalamus receives input from structures such as the basal ganglia, limbic system, and the cerebellum. The thalamus also receives input from the cerebral cortex so that feedback can be relayed. As such, the thalamus is connected to all the major areas of the brain.[7]

The hypothalamus controls important functions to everyday life, such as modulating hunger and thirst, including certain autonomic and endocrine functions. The pineal and pituitary glands are important endocrine structures that modulate many hormones in addition to helping with the sleep-wake cycle.[7]

Cerebellum

The cerebellum is located adjacent to the brain stem. This portion of the brain is primarily responsible for aiding motor function. The cerebellum does this by coordinating rapid alternating movements, balance, and position sense. Disease of the cerebellum may present with dysfunction of speech, tremor, or ocular findings, such as nystagmus.[7] Cerebellar disease may also be found with examination findings of abnormal gait, or abnormal findings on finger-to-nose or heel-shin testing.

Brain Stem

The brain stem is generally categorized into 3 structural components: medulla, pons, and midbrain. The brain stem is the most primitive portion of the brain, and is responsible for many critical neurologic functions. One example of this is the reticular formation that extends throughout the brain stem. This portion of the brain is important in controlling many critical body functions, such as breathing, blood pressure, and alertness. The brain stem is also where nearly all of the cranial nerves arise and are listed in the following sections based on anatomic location.[7]

Medulla

The medulla is the most caudal portion of the brain stem and ends at the level of the foramen magnum where the spinal cord begins. Cranial nerves (CN) that arise from this portion of the brain include the hypoglossal (CN XII), glossopharyngeal (CN IX), vagus (CN X), and portions of the accessory nerve (CN XI). The medulla also contains important neurologic pathways. Somatosensory tracts pass through the medulla and are those nerve fibers that relay peripheral sensation to the brain for interpretation. In converse, the corticospinal tracts transmit information from the cerebellum to the spinal cord and also pass through the medulla. The pyramids are a ventral structure of the medulla where the corticospinal tracts traverse the midline, decussate, and then transmit impulses to the opposite side of the body. It is the process of decussating, or crossing the midline, that results in the right or left side of the brain being responsible for sensation or movement on the opposite side of the body.[7]

Pons
The pons is located between the medulla and the midbrain. The abducens (CN VI), facial (CN VII), vestibulocochlear (CN VIII), and trigeminal nerves (CN V) are located at the level of the pons. This portion of the brain acts as a message center between the cerebellum and the cerebrum.[7]

Midbrain
The final portion of the brain stem is the midbrain. This is the most cephalic portion of the brain stem and acts primarily in coordination of eye movement in addition to reflexes associated with hearing and vision. As such, the optic (CN II), oculomotor (CN III), and trochlear nerves (CN IV) arise here.[7]

VASCULAR NEUROANATOMY

The brain requires about 20% of the body's oxygen supply and approximately 15% of the cardiac output. The circulation of the brain can be divided into anterior and posterior components. The carotid arteries give rise to the anterior circulation, and the vertebral arteries comprise the posterior circulation (**Fig. 1**). Together the anterior and posterior circulations merge to form the Circle of Willis. The Circle of Willis is a circular ring where several major blood vessels arise to provide cerebral blood flow.

Anterior Circulation

The left and right carotid arteries supply the anterior circulation of the brain. The trunk of the internal carotid travels to the Circle of Willis and divides into the middle and anterior cerebral arteries. The middle cerebral artery (MCA) supplies blood to the parietal, occipital, and temporal lobes, as well as a small portion of the frontal lobe. The lenticulostriate arteries also arise from the MCA, supply the internal capsule and basal ganglia, and are known for their nature of progressive arteriosclerosis leading to stroke. The anterior cerebral artery supplies a small area that is localized to the medial portion of the frontal and parietal lobes.[8]

Posterior Circulation

The left and right vertebral arteries primarily supply the posterior circulation of the brain; however, the anterior spinal artery also vascularizes a small segment of the brain stem. Portions of the vertebral arteries are directly responsible for feeding the most caudal portions of the brain stem. At the level where the medulla meets the pons, the vertebral arteries converge to form the basilar artery. The basilar artery provides

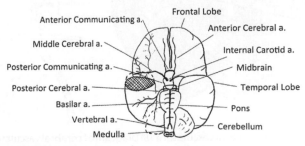

Fig. 1. Basic neuroanantomy.

circulation to the remainder of the brain stem in addition to the cerebellum. It is important to note several arteries that arise from the posterior circulation at the level of the basilar artery that supply the cerebellum, as obstruction of these arteries leads to specific clinical syndromes. Most superiorly is the superior cerebellar artery, then below is the anterior inferior cerebellar artery (AICA), and finally near the level where the vertebral arteries give rise to the basilar artery is the posterior inferior cerebellar artery (PICA). The basilar artery terminates by dividing into the left and right posterior cerebral arteries that comprise the posterior portion of the Circle of Willis and allow for communication with the anterior blood supply (**Fig. 2**).[8]

Venous Circulation

The venous circulation generally does not get as much attention as the arterial system because cerebral venous thrombosis is an uncommon form of stroke. It is important to be familiar with the venous drainage system, however, as occlusion can lead to acute stroke symptoms and significant morbidity and mortality. The superior sagittal sinus, straight sinus, and transverse sinus converge at the confluence of sinuses near the occiput. The transverse sinus communicates with the sigmoid sinus, allowing for venous drainage into the internal jugular vein.[9] Cerebral venous thrombosis is discussed later in this article, as are the common risk factors and locations for venous thrombosis.

PATHOPHYSIOLOGY

As was discussed when covering the difference between stroke types, most strokes are classified as either ischemic or hemorrhagic. The most common type of stroke is ischemic thrombotic stroke; however, low partial pressures of oxygen, hypotension, and impaired oxygen use are all additional physiologic states that can lead to ischemia and neuronal death or dysfunction. Some additional forms of stroke occur as a result of a combination of ischemia and hemorrhage.

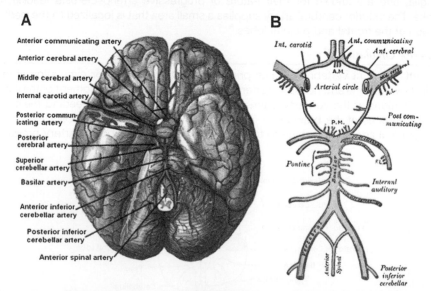

Fig. 2. Circle of Willis. (*A*) Cerebral vasculature. (*B*) Diagram of cerebral vasculature. (*Reprinted from* Gray H. Anatomy of the human body. 20th edition. Philadelphia: Lea & Febinger; 1918.)

Large Vessel Stroke

Large cerebral vessels predominantly become occluded as a result of either thrombus or embolus. Sites of localized thrombus formation within a vessel generally occur because of the nature of blood flow and anatomy. Most frequently, thrombus can form at the bifurcation of the common carotid artery where it transitions into the internal and external carotid arteries. Additional common sites for thrombus formation include the origin of the MCA, the convergence of the vertebral arteries to become the basilar artery, and the division of the basilar into the posterior portion of the Circle of Willis. All of these sites are prone to the development of arteriosclerosis because of narrowing and changes in the angles of the arising vessels.[10]

Embolisms are frequently caused by cardiac thrombi, which can be seen as a result of wall motion abnormalities after myocardial infarction, valvular disease, or irregular heart rhythms, such as atrial fibrillation. Other sources of emboli can be carotid plaques, venous thrombi that pass through structural cardiac defects, or emboli caused by fat, air, or tumor.[10]

Small Vessel Stroke

Although small vessels can also become occluded owing to the same mechanisms that generally lead to large vessel disease, smaller vessels tend to have other mechanisms for infarction. This disease is generally a result of occlusion caused by arteriosclerosis, but can also be caused by pathology, such as vasculitis. Vasculitis is frequently a result of infection, and the types of infection have changed over time. Immunosuppression has led to opportunistic infections as a more common occurrence. It is important to note that autoimmune forms of vasculitis and cerebral amyloid angiopathy also result in small vessel ischemic strokes.[10]

Hemorrhagic Stroke

Intraparenchymal hemorrhage

Spontaneous intraparenchymal hemorrhages generally present in mid to late life with peak incidence around 60 years of age.[10] Most bleeds are attributable to small vessels as a result of long-standing hypertension. Other etiologies include coagulation disorders, trauma, neoplasms, amyloid angiopathy, vasculitis, vascular malformations, and fusiform aneurysms. Bleeds that occur in the basal ganglia and thalamus are termed deep hemorrhages, whereas bleeds within the cerebral hemispheres are termed lobar hemorrhages. Bleeds within the putamen are the most common, representing 50% to 60% of intraparenchymal hemorrhages.[10]

Aneurysmal subarachnoid hemorrhages

Subarachnoid hemorrhage (SAH) accounts for approximately 5% of all stroke and is estimated to affect about 30,000 Americans annually.[11] SAH is an important disease owing to the significant mortality. In some populations, mortality rates have been documented as high as 45%, and there is significant morbidity among survivors. The most frequent cause of SAH is rupture of a saccular (berry) aneurysm. Saccular aneurysms represent the most common intracranial aneurysms.[10] The etiology of saccular aneurysms is unknown.

Within the United States, risk factors for the development of aneurysmal SAH include hypertension, smoking, and heavy alcohol abuse. Cocaine and phenylpropanolamine, both sympathomimetic agents, have been implicated as risk factors for the development of SAH. Smoking, hypertension, family history of cerebrovascular disease, and female gender (especially postmenopausal) have also been associated with the development of multiple aneurysms.[11] Several genetic syndromes, including autosomal dominant polycystic kidney disease, neurofibromatosis type 1, Marfan syndrome, and type IV Ehlers-Danlos syndrome, have been linked to aneurysm formation and subsequent rupture.[10]

Vascular Malformations

Vascular malformations significantly increase the risk for stokes. Arteriovenous malformations are the most common form of vascular malformation resulting in hemorrhage. This congenital disease is generally found between the ages of 10 and 30, with seizure or hemorrhage as the presenting symptom. These types of malformations generally arise within the subarachnoid space and are most commonly found within the posterior portions of the MCA territory. Other malformations leading to stroke include cavernous angiomas, capillary telangiectasias, and venous angiomas.[10]

Cerebral Venous Thrombosis

Cerebral venous thrombosis (CVT) is an uncommon and potentially difficult disease to diagnose. CVT has been shown to affect all age ranges and has many possible underlying risk factors. CVT is estimated to account for only 0.5% to 1.0% of all strokes.[12]

There are 2 basic mechanisms that lead to clinical findings suggestive of CVT: (1) patients who have elevated intracranial pressure (ICP) as a result of impaired venous flow and/or (2) those with focal disease from venous ischemia or hemorrhage.[12] Common signs and symptoms of CVT may include headache, papilledema, isolated elevated ICP, focal neurologic deficit, seizure, and/or encephalopathy. Other rare clinical symptoms have also been reported.[12]

Much of the data on CVT comes from a single study of 624 patients. The minimum age for enrollment was 15 years, and the mean age of the affected population was 39, which highlights the degree to which CVT affects younger patients.[13] Predisposing conditions for CVT, in order of prevalence, include but are not limited to oral contraceptives (54.3%), prothrombotic conditions (34.1%), pregnancy/puerperium (21%), and infection (12.3%).[9] There have also been specific anatomic locations that have increased incidence of disease. The most frequent locations are the superior sagittal sinus (62%), transverse sinus (41%–45%), straight sinus (18%), and cortical veins (17%).[9] The American Stroke Association (ASA), in conjunction with the AHA, has published guidelines to aid clinicians in the diagnosis and management of CVT.[9]

STROKE SYNDROMES

AIS results from loss of blood supply to a region of the brain. Occlusion of a vessel can be secondary to a thrombotic or embolic event. Rapid recognition of stroke has become of paramount importance with the increased acceptance and availability of intravenous thrombolysis for the treatment of stroke.

Embolic strokes are most commonly caused by embolization of mural thrombus (25% of ischemic strokes) secondary to myocardial infarction, atrial fibrillation, or mitral valve disease, but may also occur when clot forms at the site of an ulcerated plaque in the internal carotid artery or ascending aorta and then embolizes.[9,13] Other cardiac abnormalities predisposing to embolic strokes include patent foramen ovale, atrial septal defects, and atrial septal aneurysm.[9] Embolic events usually cause maximum deficit at onset, and frequently occur while the patient is awake.[9]

Thrombotic strokes generally occur at the site of an ulcerated plaque within a vessel. Thrombotic strokes tend to gradually reach their maximum deficit over a period of hours or days. Thrombotic strokes often occur during sleep, and the patient or family notices the deficits when the patient wakes up in the morning.[9] Risk factors for thrombotic strokes include atherosclerosis; acquired hypercoagulable states, such as pregnancy, infection, or surgery; and congenital hypercoagulable states, such as protein C and S deficiencies, antithrombin III deficiency, sickle cell disease, factor V Leiden, lupus anti-coagulant, and antiphospholipid antibodies.[9,14] Sleep-disordered breathing, such as obstructive sleep apnea, may also be a risk factor for thrombotic stroke.[15,16]

Stroke can follow occlusion of a large vessel, such as the internal carotid artery, anterior cerebral artery, middle cerebral artery, posterior cerebral artery, vertebroba-silar artery, anterior inferior cerebellar artery, posterior inferior cerebellar artery, or superior cerebellar artery (Table 2). Stroke may also be caused by the occlusion of a small penetrating artery, referred to as a lacunar infarct.

Ischemic strokes can also be divided into occlusion of anterior or posterior circulation. Anterior circulation infarcts result in frontal, temporal, and/or parietal lobe deficits, whereas posterior circulation strokes affect the occipital lobes, cerebellum, and brainstem. Less commonly, stroke can be secondary to thrombosis of an intracranial venous sinus.

Although intracranial hemorrhage may have a different clinical presentation than ischemic stroke, there is significant overlap of the clinical features. Intracranial hemor-rhage usually occurs during waking hours.[9] Intracranial hemorrhage can be classified as intraparenchymal, intraventricular, subarachnoid, subdural, or epidural, based on the location of the bleed. Because the treatment of acute ischemic stroke may include thrombolytics and antiplatelet agents, the identification of intracranial hemorrhage is paramount in differentiating between stroke types. The use of noncontrast head CT can generally exclude intraparenchymal hemorrhage, subdural hematomas, and epidural hematomas, but the exclusion of SAH may require a lumbar puncture if the

Table 2 Partial list of major stroke syndromes	
Carotid	Aphasia (dominant hemisphere) or neglect (nondominant hemisphere) Contralateral homonymous hemianopsia Contralateral motor/sensory loss of face, arm, and leg Conjugate ipsilateral eye deviation
MCA	Aphasia (dominant hemisphere) or neglect (nondominant hemisphere) Contralateral homonymous hemianopsia Contralateral motor/sensory loss face/arm > leg
ACA	Apathy, abulia, disinhibition Conjugate eye deviation Contralateral motor/sensory loss leg > arm
PICA	Ipsilateral palatal weakness, Horner syndrome Wallenberg syndrome Ipsilateral limb ataxia Decreased pain/temperature contralateral body
AICA	Ipsilateral deafness Ipsilateral facial motor/sensory loss Ipsilateral limb ataxia Decreased pain/temperature contralateral body
Basilar	Altered consciousness Oculomotor difficulties, facial paresis Ataxia, quadriparesis

Abbreviations: ACA, anterior cerebral artery, AICA, anterior inferior cerebellar artery; MCA, middle cerebral artery; PICA, posterior inferior cerebellar artery.
Data from Goetz CG. Textbook of clinical neurology. 3rd edition. Philadelphia: Elsevier; 2007; and Goldstein JN, Greer DM. Rapid focused neurologic assessment in the emergency department and ICU. Emerg Med Clin North Am 2009;27(1):5.

noncontrast head CT is negative. CT scanning has a sensitivity of 91% to 98% for identifying SAH, and the sensitivity decreases with time.[14] A recent study suggests sensitivity of 100% (97%–100%) if CT scanning is performed within 6 hours of symptom onset.[17] The clinical presentation of SAH is usually different from that of an ischemic stroke. Classically, SAH presents as the sudden onset of a severe headache. The presence of SAH mandates a search for an aneurysm or arteriovenous malformation within the circulation of the brain. Risk factors for intracranial hemorrhage include hypertension, trauma, anticoagulant medications, coagulopathies, stimulant drugs (cocaine and amphetamines), amyloidosis, and brain tumors.[9] Identification and treatment of intracranial hemorrhage is discussed in detail in the article by Caceres and Goldstein elsewhere in this issue.

Carotid Artery Occlusion

Carotid artery occlusion presents with aphasia if the dominant hemisphere is involved and contralateral neglect if the nondominant hemisphere is affected. There is motor and sensory loss of the face, arm, and leg on the opposite side from the occlusion. The eyes will deviate toward the side of the occlusion, and there may be a visual field deficit on the side opposite from the occluded carotid artery.[18]

Middle Cerebral Artery Occlusion

Occlusion of the MCA will cause global aphasia, if the occlusion occurs in the dominant hemisphere, and contralateral hemispatial neglect, if it occurs in the nondominant hemisphere. Most right-handed people and 70% to 80% of left-handed people have their language centers in the left hemisphere.[18] There will be motor and sensory deficits of the side opposite to the occlusion, involving the face and arm, and to a lesser extent, the leg. There may be a homonymous hemianopia, and conjugate eye deviation toward the side of the lesion.[9]

The MCA divides into superior and inferior divisions. The superior division within the dominant hemisphere supplies the Broca area in the frontal lobe, ischemia of which is responsible for motor aphasia. With Broca aphasia, speech will be halting and poorly articulated.[9] The inferior division of the MCA supplies the Wernicke area in the temporal lobe, ischemia of which causes sensory aphasia. With Wernicke aphasia, speech is fluent but incorrect words and nonsense words may be present, making it difficult to understand the meaning that the speaker is trying to convey.[9]

Anterior Cerebral Artery Occlusion

Occlusion of the anterior cerebral artery will classically cause contralateral motor and sensory deficits, more prominent in the leg than the arm. The face and tongue are usually spared.[19] Lack of concern and disinhibition are frequently present. Incontinence may be present, as well as primitive frontal lobe reflexes (grasp and suck).[9]

Posterior Cerebral Artery Occlusion

Posterior cerebral artery infarcts most commonly occur secondary to embolization.[19] Posterior cerebral artery occlusion frequently presents with a contralateral visual field cut in the form of a homonymous hemianopia. Visual agnosia may be present, as well as disorders of reading, if the PCA occlusion is in the left (dominant) hemisphere.[19] Alexia (inability to read words and sentences) with or without agraphia (inability to write and spell) may be present.[19] Prosopagnosia, or the inability to recognize faces, may also occur with posterior cerebral artery occlusion. There is usually no paralysis. Sensory loss may be present or absent. Aphasia will not be present. Bilateral posterior cerebral artery occlusion may cause blindness.[9,20] Bilateral posterior cerebral artery occlusions may also cause permanent amnesia, with the inability to form new memories.[19]

Superior Cerebellar Artery Occlusion

Superior cerebellar artery occlusion may classically present with ipsilateral limb dysmetria, ipsilateral Horner syndrome, contralateral loss of pain and temperature sensation, and contralateral weakness of the fourth cranial nerve.[19] This classic presentation is not commonly seen, however.[19]

Posterior Inferior Cerebellar Artery Occlusion

Posterior inferior cerebellar infarcts are the most frequently encountered cerebellar strokes.[19] PICA obstruction may lead to the lateral medullary syndrome (Wallenberg syndrome), consisting of decreased pain and temperature sensation of the ipsilateral face and contralateral trunk and extremities (because of damage to the spinothalamic tract). Other deficits caused by PICA occlusion include Horner syndrome (ipsilateral ptosis, miosis, and anhydrosis), dysphagia, ipsilateral limb ataxia, nystagmus, diplopia, and myoclonus of the ipsilateral palate. These patients are at risk for aspiration.[21]

Anterior Inferior Cerebellar Artery Occlusion

AICA occlusion may present as sudden deafness owing to ischemia of the inner ear causing cochlear dysfunction.[22] AICA occlusion classically presets with vertigo, vomiting, tinnitus, and dysarthria.[19] AICA stroke also causes ipsilateral facial weakness and ipsilateral limb ataxia. Owing to ischemia of the spinothalamic tract, contralateral pain and temperature sensation may be impaired.[18,23]

Vertebrobasilar Artery Occlusion

High-grade occlusion of the vertebrobasilar system causes loss of circulation to the cerebellum, brain stem, thalamus, and occipital lobe. The result is frequently death or major disability, such as coma, quadriplegia, ataxia, dysarthria, cranial nerve dysfunction, and visual deficits.[24] Rarely, basilar artery thrombosis may cause "locked-in syndrome," in which the patient cannot move or speak but cognition remains intact.[19,24]

Lacunar Infarcts

A lacunar infarct results from occlusion of a deep penetrating artery. These small-vessel occlusions account for 25% of all ischemic strokes. Depending on the region supplied by the occluded penetrating artery, the neurologic findings vary. Lacunar infarcts may present as pure motor hemiparesis, involving the posterior limb of the internal capsule. This syndrome may present as paresis of unilateral face, arm, and leg without sensory findings. Another presentation is ataxic hemiparesis, involving the internal capsule and corona radiata. This syndrome generally will cause ataxia and weakness of one leg. Dysarthria/clumsy hand results from a lacunar infarct involving the pons or internal capsule. This syndrome consists of slurred speech and weakness of one arm. A lacunar infarct in the thalamus may cause a pure sensory stroke. This syndrome will usually cause diminished sensation of unilateral face, arm, and leg. A mixed sensorimotor stroke may result from a lacunar infarct in the thalamus and internal capsule.[9,25,26]

Border Zone Infarction Syndromes

Watershed strokes, or border zone infarction syndromes, generally follow periods during which systemic oxygen delivery is impaired, such as with hypoxia or hypotension. There are a variety of different syndromes attributable to border zone infarction. Anterior border zone infarction syndrome may consist of aphasia and proximal arm weakness, or motor weakness in the lower leg.[9,19] Posterior border zone infarction may cause visual disturbances, such as lateral homonymous hemianopia.[19]

Cerebral Venous Thrombosis

An uncommon cause of cerebral infarction is thrombosis of one of the venous sinuses in the brain. CVT may present as headache, with or without cranial nerve palsies. More severely affected patients may present with seizures and/or coma. Papilledema is frequently present. The incidence of this entity is rising, as it is being recognized more frequently as a result of newer imaging modalities, including CT angiography (CTA) and MRI/MR angiography.[27] The 2011 AHA/ASA statement for physicians on the diagnosis and management of CVT discusses the benefits of CT and CT venogram (CTV) versus MRI and MR venogram (MRV). In summary, CT with CTV is the test of choice in the acute phase of thrombosis. It is noted that MRI and MRV are more sensitive after the acute phase of thrombosis, but the article discusses additional strengths and weakness of each test when used to diagnose CVT.[9]

DEMOGRAPHICS AND RISK FACTORS FOR ISCHEMIC STROKE

Stroke remains the third leading cause of death in the United States, causing 137,000 deaths annually.[28] Age older than 55 is considered a risk factor for stroke, with doubling of the risk for stroke with each decade over age 55.[28] The aging of the US population has contributed significantly to the growth in number of emergency department visits in the United States, with a 19% increase in overall visits from 1995 to 2005, yet the increase in visits by patients aged 65 to 74 was 34% over a similar period.[29] It is anticipated that the aging of the US population will lead to an increase in the number of strokes presenting to emergency departments in the coming years.[28] There is also literature to suggest that strokes are not uncommon in younger patients, and that 10% of all strokes occur in people younger than 50.[30,31] In fact, in a recent prospective study in Switzerland, 14% of strokes over a 6-year period occurred in patients younger than 46 years.[32] Other risk factors for stroke include diabetes, hypertension, hyperlipidemia, smoking, obesity, atrial fibrillation, recent myocardial infarction, sickle cell anemia, vasculitides, fibromuscular dysplasia, and family history.[30,33–36] Recent herpes zoster infection, especially herpes zoster ophthalmicus, may also be a risk factor for stroke.[37]

The epidemic of obesity, diabetes, and hypertension among young Americans may lead to an increase in the incidence of stroke in young people.[38] In addition to the traditional risk factors stated previously, additional risk factors for stroke in people younger than 50 include patent foramen ovale, atrial septal defect, dissection of carotid or vertebral arteries, hypercoaguability, and autoimmune disorders.[31,32] Oral contraceptives, pregnancy, mitral valve prolapse, homocystinuria, polycystic ovary syndrome, cigarette smoking, binge alcohol drinking, and cocaine and amphetamine use may also predispose to stroke in young adults.[9,39,40] In addition to acute ischemic stroke, cocaine and amphetamines may predispose young people to SAH and intracerebral hemorrhage.[9]

Another important cause of stroke in young adults is carotid artery dissection. Carotid artery dissection may be spontaneous or traumatic. Patients with carotid dissection may present with Horner syndrome owing to loss of sympathetic innervation within the carotid sheath. Patients may present with isolated neck pain, and trauma causing dissection may be minimal.[9]

In summary, stroke is a frequent and time-sensitive emergency department presentation. Rapid identification, imaging, neurologic consultation, and treatment of stroke are essential. Knowledge of the basic neuroanatomy, clinical presentation, and CT findings of various stroke syndromes and hemorrhage aid the emergency physician in diagnosis and management. Application of the NIHSS score (**Table 1**) will allow the emergency physician, in consultation with a neurologist, to administer thrombolytic therapy when appropriate.[41]

REFERENCES

1. Goldstein LB, Bushnell CD, Adams RJ, et al. Guidelines for the primary prevention of stroke: a guideline for healthcare professionals from the American Heart Association/American Stroke Association. Stroke 2010;42:517–84.
2. Cruz-Flores S, Rabinstein A, Biller J, et al. Racial-ethnic disparities in stroke care: the American experience: a statement for healthcare professionals from the American Heart Association/American Stroke Association. Stroke 2011;42(7):2091–116.
3. Roach ES, Golomb MR, Adams R, et al. Management of stroke in infants and children: a scientific statement from a special writing group of the American Heart Association Stroke Council and the Council on Cardiovascular Disease in the Young. Stroke 2008;39(9):2644–91.
4. Task Force Members, Schwamm LH, Pancioli A, Acker JE 3rd, et al. Recommendations for the establishment of stroke systems of care: recommendations from the American Stroke Association's Task Force on the Development of Stroke Systems. Stroke 2005;36(3):690–703.
5. Alberts MJ, Latchaw RE, Selman WR, et al. Recommendations for comprehensive stroke centers: a consensus statement from the brain attack coalition. Stroke 2005;36(7):1597–616.
6. Easton JD, Saver JL, Albers GW, et al. Definition and evaluation of transient ischemic attack: a scientific statement for healthcare professionals from the American Heart Association/American Stroke Association Stroke Council; Council on Cardiovascular Surgery and Anesthesia; Council on Cardiovascular Radiology and Intervention; Council on Cardiovascular Nursing; and the Interdisciplinary Council on Peripheral Vascular Disease: the American Academy of Neurology affirms the value of this statement as an educational tool for neurologists. Stroke 2009;40:2276–93.
7. Silverthorn D. Human physiology: an integrated approach. 4th edition. San Francisco (CA): Pearson/Benjamin Cummings; 2007.
8. Gilman S. Manter and Gatz's essentials of clinical neuroanatomy and neurophysiology. 9th edition. Philadelphia: F.A. Davis; 1996.
9. Saposnik G, Barinagarrementeria F, Brown RD, et al. Diagnosis and management of cerebral venous thrombosis: a statement for healthcare professionals from the American Heart Association/American Stroke Association. Stroke 2011;42:1158–92.
10. Kumar V. Robbins and Cotran pathologic basis of disease. 7th edition. Philadelphia: Elsevier Saunders; 2005.
11. Bederson JB, Connolly ES, Batjer HH, et al. Guidelines for the management of aneurysmal subarachnoid hemorrhage: a statement for healthcare professionals from a special writing group of the stroke council, American Heart Association. Stroke 2009;40:994–1025.
12. Bousser MG, Ferro JM. Cerebral venous thrombosis: an update. Lancet Neurol 2007;6(2):162–70.
13. Ferro JM. Prognosis of cerebral vein and dural sinus thrombosis: results of the International Study on Cerebral Vein and Dural Sinus Thrombosis (ISCVT). Stroke 2004;35(3):664–70.

14. Marques MA, Murad FF, Ristow AV, et al. Acute carotid occlusion and stroke due to antiphospholipid antibody syndrome: case report and literature review. Int Angiol 2010;29(4):380–4.
15. Johnson KG, Johnson DC. Frequency of sleep apnea in stroke and TIA patients: a meta-analysis. J Clin Sleep Med 2010;6(2):131–7.
16. Ramar K, Surani S. The relationship between sleep disorders and stroke. Postgrad Med 2010;122(6):145–53.
17. Perry JJ, Stiell IG, Sivilotti MLA, et al. Sensitivity of computed tomography performed within six hours of onset of headache for diagnosis of subarachnoid haemorrhage: prospective cohort study. BMJ 2011;343:d4277.
18. Goldstein JN, Greer DM. Rapid focused neurological assessment in the emergency department and ICU. Emerg Med Clin North Am 2009;27(1):1–16, vii.
19. Bogousslavsky J, Caplan LR. Stroke syndromes. Cambridge (United Kingdom); New York: Cambridge University Press; 2001.
20. Helseth E. Posterior cerebral artery stroke. Medscape Reference. March 29, 2011.
21. Khedr EM, Abo-Elfetoh N. Therapeutic role of rTMS on recovery of dysphagia in patients with lateral medullary syndrome and brainstem infarction. J Neurol Neurosurg Psychiatr 2010;81(5):495–9.
22. Lee H, Sohn SI, Jung DK, et al. Sudden deafness and anterior inferior cerebellar artery infarction. Stroke 2002;33(12):2807–12.
23. Lee H, Cho YW. Auditory disturbance as a prodrome of anterior inferior cerebellar artery infarction. J Neurol Neurosurg Psychiatr 2003;74(12):1644–8.
24. Kaye V. Vertebrobasilar stroke. Medscape Reference. March 29, 2011.
25. Sacco S, Marini C, Totaro R, et al. A population-based study of the incidence and prognosis of lacunar stroke. Neurology 2006;66(9):1335–8.
26. Papamitsakis N. Lacunar syndromes. Medscape Reference. December 10, 2011.
27. Lipton RB, Silberstein SD, Dalessio DJ. Wolff's headache and other pain. New York; Oxford (United Kingdom): Oxford University Press; 2001.
28. Fonarow GC, Reeves MJ, Zhao X, et al. Age-related differences in characteristics, performance measures, treatment trends, and outcomes in patients with ischemic stroke. Circulation 2010;121(7):879–91.
29. Xu KT, Nelson BK, Berk S. The changing profile of patients who used emergency department services in the United States: 1996 to 2005. Ann Emerg Med 2009; 54(6):805.e1-7–10.e1-7.
30. De Silva R, Gamage R, Wewelwala C, et al. Young strokes in Sri Lanka: an unsolved problem. J Stroke Cerebrovasc Dis 2009;18(4):304–8.
31. Janssen AWM, de Leeuw FE, Janssen MCH. Risk factors for ischemic stroke and transient ischemic attack in patients under age 50. J Thromb Thrombolysis 2011; 31(1):85–91.
32. Arnold M, Halpern M, Meier N, et al. Age-dependent differences in demographics, risk factors, co-morbidity, etiology, management, and clinical outcome of acute ischemic stroke. J Neurol 2008;255(10):1503–7.
33. Marx JA, Hockberger RS, Walls RM, et al. Rosen's emergency medicine: concepts and clinical practice. Philadelphia: Mosby/Elsevier; 2010.
34. Rae-Grant A, Weiner HL. Weiner and Levitt's neurology. Philadelphia: Lippincott Williams & Wilkins; 2008.
35. Bosnar-Puretić M, Basić-Kes V, Jurasić MJ, et al. The association of obesity and cerebrovascular disease in young adults—a pilot study. Acta Clin Croat 2009;48(3):295–8.
36. Jood K, Ladenvall C, Rosengren A, et al. Family history in ischemic stroke before 70 years of age: the Sahlgrenska Academy Study on Ischemic Stroke. Stroke 2005;36(7):1383–7.

37. Kang JH, Ho JD, Chen YH, et al. Increased risk of stroke after a herpes zoster attack: a population-based follow-up study. Stroke 2009;40(11):3443–8.
38. Kitzman-Ulrich H, Wilson DK, St George SM, et al. The integration of a family systems approach for understanding youth obesity, physical activity, and dietary programs. Clin Child Fam Psychol Rev 2010;13(3):231–53.
39. Parlakgumus HA, Haydardedeoglu B. A review of cardiovascular complications of pregnancy. Ginekol Pol 2010;81(4):292–7.
40. de Groot PC, Dekkers OM, Romijn JA, et al. PCOS, coronary heart disease, stroke and the influence of obesity: a systematic review and meta-analysis. Hum Reprod Update 2011;17(4):495–500.
41. Akins PT, Delemos C, Wentworth D, et al. Can emergency department physicians safely and effectively initiate thrombolysis for acute ischemic stroke? Neurology 2000;55(12):1801–5.

Prehospital Diagnosis and Management of Patients with Acute Stroke

Ricky Kue, MD, MPH, FACEP[a,b,*], Alaina Steck, MD, FACEP[b]

KEYWORDS

- Acute stroke • Management • Prehospital diagnosis • Ischemic stroke

KEY POINTS

- Significant advances in the early management of ischemic stroke have been made since the original 1995 publication of the National Institute of Neurologic Disorders and Stroke.
- One concept in stroke care that has become better understood in these past few years is the importance of time management and the ability to deliver patients with acute stroke to appropriate care as soon as possible.
- The key factors for prehospital care include the following: early identification of suspected stroke symptoms, early activation of emergency medical services, immediate and focused medical interventions to reduce secondary cerebral injuries, timely initiation of transportation, and rapid notification of appropriate receiving facilities capable of managing patients with stroke.
- Despite this increased time window for therapy, minimizing any delay to definitive therapy remains the current focus in the prehospital phase of stroke care.

Significant advances in the early management of ischemic stroke have been made since the original 1995 publication of the National Institute of Neurologic Disorders and Stroke (NINDS) data demonstrated the benefit of early intravenous administration of tissue plasminogen activator (t-PA) to select patients with acute ischemic stroke within a 3-hour onset window of suspected stroke symptoms.[1] One concept in stroke care that has become better understood in these past few years is the importance of time management and the ability to deliver patients with acute stroke to appropriate care as soon as possible. When considering the prehospital phase of stroke care as the time interval before arrival to an appropriate receiving hospital, one must consider several factors, such as the early identification of suspected stroke symptoms by both

a Boston Emergency Medical Services, Office of Research, Training and Quality Improvement, 785 Albany Street, Boston, MA 02118, USA; b Department of Emergency Medicine, Boston University School of Medicine, 1 Boston Medical Center Place, Dowling 1 South, Boston, MA 02118, USA
* Corresponding author. Boston Emergency Medical Services, Office of Research, Training, and Quality Improvement, 785 Albany Street, Boston, MA 02118.
E-mail address: kue@bostonems.org

Emerg Med Clin N Am 30 (2012) 617–635
doi:10.1016/j.emc.2012.05.003
0733-8627/12/$ – see front matter © 2012 Elsevier Inc. All rights reserved.

the public and health care providers, early activation of emergency medical services (EMS), immediate and focused medical interventions to reduce secondary cerebral injuries, timely initiation of transportation, and rapid notification of appropriate receiving facilities capable of managing patients with stroke. Similar to current criteria for transport to a trauma center or primary coronary catheterization centers for ST-elevation myocardial infarctions, a robust EMS system will also take into consideration which destination hospital has the resources to appropriately manage patients with acute stroke. The American Heart Association (AHA) and the American Stroke Association (ASA) have extended its current treatment guideline for fibrinolytic administration to 4.5 hours of onset of stroke symptoms because of the recent prospective studies.[2–4] Despite this increased time window for therapy, minimizing any delay to definitive therapy remains the current focus in the prehospital phase of stroke care.

BACKGROUND

In the United States, ischemic stroke continues to be the third leading cause of death in adults and affects approximately 700,000 individuals annually.[5] The prehospital phase of acute stroke management encompasses all aspects of care before the arrival at a medical treatment facility. Although typically associated with EMS care, this phase also includes aspects related to the general public. Specifically, it is important that the public quickly identifies symptoms so that the activation of the EMS system occurs as soon as possible. Based on data from the Paul Coverdell National Acute Stroke Registry analyzed by the Centers for Disease Control and Prevention, it is estimated that fewer than half (48%) of the patients with stroke for whom symptom onset data was available arrived at the emergency department (ED) within 2 hours of symptom onset and prehospital delays were shorter for patients transported to the ED by ambulance compared with those who did not receive ambulance transport. The interval between ED arrival and brain imaging was also significantly reduced for those arriving by ambulance.[6] These findings suggest a need for extensive public education about stroke symptom awareness and early activation of EMS and highlight the need to improve the way EMS processes patients with stroke so that any unnecessary delays to intervention are avoided.

In an effort to improve overall stroke care, the concept of a stroke chain of recovery is used as a model for reducing delays to stroke intervention akin to other similar concepts, such as the trauma golden hour or time-is-muscle concept in acute coronary care.[7,8] The chain-of-recovery concept describes 5 distinct components: (1) identification of the patient with the stroke, (2) dispatch system by 911 activation, (3) EMS provider factors, (4) alert to ED and stroke specialists, and (5) diagnosis and treatment. The goal of this article is to examine the different prehospital components that impact the overall time to definitive stroke care and to discuss strategies that have helped make the delivery of prehospital stroke care more efficient.

COMMUNITY AWARENESS AND EDUCATION

A previous review of prehospital stroke care[9] noted that public understanding and education remains the weakest link in the chain of recovery. Although EMS efforts to minimize scene time and optimize disposition and transport are a fundamental link in efficient and effective prehospital care, the factor that has been consistently shown to have the biggest impact on symptom-onset-to-arrival time is public awareness, not only of stroke signs and symptoms but also of the need to call EMS for transport rather than to provide private transportation to the treating facility.[9–11] A 1999 study of patients with acute stroke demonstrated that lower socioeconomic status, education level, not calling EMS, and living alone were factors associated with later presentation to the ED.[12] Another study demonstrated similar findings whereby the reduction in time to ED presentation was typically associated with the Caucasian race and activation of EMS. In this case series, approximately 40% of the patients with stroke stated that medical attention was encouraged by a friend or family member and they themselves did not call EMS.[13] Furthermore, studies have consistently shown that the time between symptom onset and the time at which a patient makes medical contact, whether by calling 911, calling a doctor, or walking in for evaluation at a medical facility, is the greatest contributor to prehospital delays.[10,14] A study published in 2000 demonstrated that even patients and bystanders who had a working knowledge of stroke warning signs did not understand the importance of notifying EMS for transport once symptoms occurred.[15] A 2005 survey in the Czech Republic found that 69% of laypersons identified stroke as a serious condition but 26% did not know what stroke was. Of those respondents who were able to identify symptoms of a stroke, only 27% would choose to call an ambulance and 10% would wait a day to see if the symptoms resolved before taking further action.[16] Additionally, a significant number of people did not understand stroke to be a treatable condition (43%). These researchers later examined the impact of a 4-year public awareness campaign on the ability of the lay public to identify stroke and then notify EMS. Unfortunately, there was no global improvement in these metrics, although respondents who did recall noticing the educational campaign performed slightly better in recognizing cerebrovascular accident (CVA) symptoms and remembering to call EMS than respondents who did not recall exposure to any educational materials.[17] Similar findings were independently uncovered in a German study in which the number of people who would seek emergency care did not change (81% vs 82%) after an intensive 3-month public awareness campaign.[18]

Efforts to increase public awareness of the symptoms of acute stroke and understanding the need for rapid EMS activation are essential. A recent German population study sought to identify the most appropriate channels for public education; respondents most frequently identified mass media (82%), family or friends (45%), and physicians (20%) as their primary sources for information about stroke.[19] There have also been several studies aimed at identifying the factors that prompt patients to call EMS. Gross muscle weakness,[9] sudden unilateral weakness, and speech difficulties are the stroke symptoms most consistently recognized by laypersons, whereas symptoms, such as dizziness/vertigo and sudden severe headache, are less frequently appreciated to be symptoms suspicious for stroke.[10] A separate study found that the most commonly recognized symptoms (weakness, altered mental status, speech changes) are also more likely to prompt patients to call 911 rather than to transport themselves to a hospital.[20] Once a patient or bystander identified symptoms, those most likely to call EMS are older, have greater preexisting disability, have more severe symptoms (as later quantified in the hospital by the National Institutes of Health Stroke Scale [NIHSS]), or have symptoms that began in the presence of bystanders.[21]

Surprisingly, stroke recognition and initial management must be emphasized even at the physician level. A German study published in 2007 found that although most primary care physicians identified stroke and transient ischemic attack (TIA) as medical emergencies (95% and 85% respectively), only two-thirds of these providers (66%–69%) would send patients with clear stroke symptoms to a hospital as an emergency referral.[22] Ensuring both public and provider awareness must be a priority if there is to be ongoing improvement in prehospital stroke care.

Community education remains a cornerstone of early stroke identification and an integral component to any program aimed at reducing prehospital delays to ED presentation. Bystander-witnessed stroke symptoms are associated with reduced time to ED presentation compared with patient self-recognition of symptoms.[23] It is important that *all* people have an understanding of stroke symptoms because it is a bystander or family member in most cases who will recognize these symptoms in a patient and activate the EMS system. One approach to improving early recognition of stroke symptoms examined stroke awareness programs designed for children in homes and communities with those at the highest risk for stroke.[11] A recent study looked at whether elementary school children in an inner-city population of New York City could be educated on stroke symptoms using contemporary music as an approach.[24] There was good success in post-training knowledge and retention of knowledge at 3 months. Another study examined the use of stroke scales designed for EMS use among the general public. A 2005 study examined using the Cincinnati Prehospital Stroke Scale as a way for the public to determine the likelihood of on-going symptoms to suggest an acute stroke. Researchers found that the general public could administer the test correctly 98% of the time and accurately relay this information to first responders and dispatchers.[25]

EMS DISPATCH AND RESPONSE

Of equal importance to the recognition of stroke symptoms and the activation of the EMS system is the ability for EMS dispatch systems to recognize the presence of an evolving stroke and immediately dispatch appropriate resources. If the message and time-urgent nature is not communicated to responding crews early on, time is lost and the window for time-critical intervention narrows. A key component to dispatch is the awareness level and education of the public to recognize and properly convey concerns of an on-going stroke to dispatch personnel. A 1995 study on a 2-tiered EMS system showed their dispatchers correctly identifying stroke in only 52% of cases based on the caller description compared with 72% in that system's paramedic providers. EMS was typically dispatched to the scene for diagnoses other than stroke.[26] Studies continue to highlight the disparities between dispatcher and EMS-provider agreement in stroke presentation as compared with other providers, such as emergency physicians.[27] Several previous studies highlight the challenges faced by dispatchers when trying to decipher whether an acute stroke is occurring: acute stroke was correctly identified at a low rate, incidents were often assigned lower acuity than was appropriate, and dispatchers had difficulty identifying certain nonspecific symptoms, such as impaired communication, weakness, or the inability to stand or walk, as symptoms suggestive of stroke.[9]

The importance of early stroke identification by EMS dispatchers cannot be overstated. A reduction in median prehospital run time to ED presentation has been shown when there is concordance between dispatcher and paramedic-provider identification of patients with stroke.[28] Although the diagnosis of a suspected stroke remains challenging even when in direct contact with patients, there remains significant room for improvement in the emergency medical dispatcher (EMD) recognition of stroke. The current EMD curriculum requires 24 hours of instruction without specific training on recognizing the warning signs of stroke. A 2005 study noted that despite the explicit use of the word stroke by callers in nearly half of the cases reviewed, the EMDs categorized only one-third (31%) of calls as suspected stroke.[29] More recent reviews have demonstrated wide variations in the sensitivity and specificity of EMD stroke identification, although the overall performance remains poor. Ellison and colleagues[27] found that EMDs in the Kansas City, Missouri EMS system had only 61% sensitivity and 20% specificity for stroke identification. In Los Angeles, EMDs identified fewer than 50% of patients with a final diagnosis of stroke, even when using the standardized Medical Priority Dispatch System algorithm (card 28: stroke/CVA), which is used in EMS systems across the United States. In this same study, EMDs had a sensitivity of 41% and specificity of 96% for the classification of acute stroke.[30]

To improve and standardize the EMD approach to identify stroke victims, a current study is ongoing to prospectively compare previous editions of proprietary dispatch instruction cards for stroke with a new diagnostic tool incorporated into the current standard dispatch instructions. This prospective trial started in 2011 and the results will help determine if the incorporation of a standard stroke-scale tool improves dispatch identification.[31] Ongoing efforts to improve EMD's role in acute stroke care should not be limited to the identification of and appropriate dispatch for stroke symptoms. EMDs also have the opportunity to facilitate prehospital care by not only gathering pertinent information (eg, time of onset) but also by administering prearrival instructions to callers (eg, to gather medication lists, avoid fall risks).

EMS IDENTIFICATION OF ACUTE STROKE

Stroke programs across the country have realized the importance of considering EMS factors as part of the overall plan to reduce time to acute stroke intervention. Prehospital factors in overall stroke management play a significant part in the overall time to presentation to a stroke treatment facility. Previous recommendations included a window to intravenous t-PA therapy within 3 hours of symptoms onset, which recently has been increased to 4.5 hours.[1,2] This change in recommendation should not be viewed only as an opportunity to increase potential treatment recipients by simply increasing the therapeutic window; rather, planning should continue to focus on reducing overall time to definitive care regardless of window length.

In 1999, Crocco and colleagues[32] examined the education and training of EMS providers in stroke recognition and knowledge. A randomly distributed survey to EMS providers from the National Registry of Emergency Medical Technicians database showed that although most providers at the paramedic and intermediate levels were knowledgeable about the signs and symptoms of acute stroke, significantly fewer could properly define a TIA or appreciate the recommended therapeutic treatment window for t-PA. Additionally, they found that EMS providers did not appreciate the importance of avoiding blood pressure reduction in patients with acute stroke.

Although it can be challenging in the EMS environment to accurately diagnose every patient encounter, it is important that those patients most likely suffering from a stroke be identified as soon and as accurately as possible so that appropriate downstream actions can be instituted. There have been many tools developed for EMS providers to increase their accuracy in diagnosing potential patients with stroke to help differentiate between patients experiencing a possible stroke versus other mimic conditions, such as vertigo or syncope. The NIHSS developed in 1983 with the NINDS group provides an accurate and standardized approach to the evaluation of stroke symptoms and severity with good inter-rater reliability.[33] The NIHSS is a multiple-item assessment tool designed for serial neurologic examination in patients with an ischemic or hemorrhagic stroke. Despite these strengths, the lengthy nature of the NIHSS and lack of consistent use by EMS providers with limited patient contact time in the prehospital phase challenges the validity of its use in this environment.[34]

Described in 1997, the Cincinnati Prehospital Stroke Scale (CPSS) is a simple 3-item scale based on the NIHSS designed specifically for EMS use. It focuses on the presence of facial palsy, arm motor weakness, and dysarthria (**Box 1**). The presence of all 3 components identified 100% of the patients with stroke.[35] When the CPSS was classically associated with secondary brain insults include severe and sustained hypoxia, hypotension, and hypoglycemia. Patients experiencing a stroke can develop airway compromise caused by decreased levels of consciousness from brainstem involvement or loss of protective reflexes. Appropriate airway monitoring for the need of intubation and early intubation to secure an unstable airway may be needed to prevent hypoxia.

The management of blood pressure (BP), both hypertension and hypotension, is an important element in the care of patients with acute stroke. Published best-practice guidelines on early stroke management are available to clinicians through the AHA/ASA scientific statement on the early management of acute ischemic stroke.[44]

Hypotension is not commonly seen after acute ischemic stroke and typically warrants a search by the clinician for a concurrent pathologic process, such as abdominal aneurysm, aortic dissection, volume depletion, decreased cardiac output, and so forth. Stroke symptoms in such a scenario would suggest a cerebral low-flow state as seen with watershed infarcts. Poststroke hypotension has been described and has been associated with worse patient outcomes, with as much as a 17.9% increase in early death for every 10–mm Hg systolic BP decrease less than 150 mm Hg.[45] Additionally, rates of neurologic worsening, poor neurologic outcomes, or death increased when the baseline systolic BP was less than 100 mm Hg or the diastolic BP was less than 70 mm Hg.

Arterial hypertension is more common with ischemic stroke presentation. Hypertension may provide appropriate cerebral perfusion pressure to an ischemic brain; however, the need for cerebral perfusion must be balanced with the known risks of hypertension-induced cerebral edema, hemorrhagic transformation of the infarct, and further vascular damage. In one study, for every 10–mm Hg increase more than 180 mm Hg in the systolic BP, the risk of neurologic deterioration increased by 40% and the risk of poor outcome increased by 23%.[46,47] In many cases, arterial BP will spontaneously trend toward normal levels within the first few hours of a stroke. Given the controversy in the treatment of arterial hypertension with patients with ischemic stroke, current guidelines do not call for routine intervention for mild to moderate arterial hypertension. The current ASA guidelines suggest the pharmacologic lowering of BP when the systolic BP is more than 220 mm Hg or the diastolic BP is more than 120 mm Hg. Currently, use of t-PA is contraindicated if pretreatment BP is greater than 185/110, which indicates a likely need for antihypertensive treatment in patients whose only disqualifying factor for t-PA treatment is the BP reading. Permissive hypertension up to 220/120 should be allowed for patients unless they are going to be given t-PA or a hemorrhagic stroke is found. EMS providers should not institute BP management in these patients unless they have prolonged transport times or are transporting patients between stroke centers and have formal physician recommendations based on diagnosis.[44] The agents for use depend greatly on the antihypertensive agents that are available to the EMS agency but typically include beta-blockers, such as labetalol or esmolol; angiotensin converting enzyme inhibitors, such as enalapril or enalaprilat; or calcium channel blockers, such as nicardipine. Vasodilator medications, such as intravenous nitrates, should be avoided because these medications can result in venous dilation and may worsen intracranial edema and pressure.

Intravenous fluids should be avoided unless there is concern for volume loss and resultant hypotension because excess intravenous fluids can result in worsening cerebral edema and subsequent brain injury. Fluids for the purpose of resuscitation should be restricted to isotonic saline to minimize any possibility of osmotic fluid shifts. Controversy remains over the use of hypertonic saline in the setting of increased intracranial pressure caused by brain edema. There are data supporting the use of hypertonic saline for this purpose[48]; however, a randomized prehospital study assessing its use did not show any benefit to patients with head injuries.[49] It is unclear how this therapy would benefit patients with ischemic stroke and remains controversial until more comparative data become available.[50]

Dextrose-containing fluid can be considered, especially when hypoglycemia is present. Hypoglycemia is a well-known stroke mimic, and glucose is the ideal substrate for neuronal cellular metabolism; thus, hypoglycemia should be avoided and corrected when present. On the other hand, hyperglycemia is detected in approximately one-third of patients with stroke on admission.[44] Hyperglycemia can promote fluid shifts across the blood-brain barrier, increase the risk of cerebral edema, and increase the risk of hemorrhagic transformation of an ischemic stroke. Blood glucose elevation can be caused by underlying diabetes mellitus, a risk factor for stroke development, but may also reflect a stress response caused by the stroke itself in nondiabetic patients. One study showed that persistent hyperglycemia more than 200 mg/dL during the first 24 hours after stroke independently predicted the expansion of the volume of ischemic stroke and poor neurologic outcomes.[51] The current stroke guidelines recommend maintaining blood glucose within a range of 80 to 140 mg/dL. Prehospital treatment of hyperglycemia will depend on local protocols. Most municipal EMS agencies do not typically include treatment options, such as insulin therapy for hyperglycemia. As discussed previously, large volumes of intravenous fluid should be avoided when managing hyperglycemia because of the possibility of cerebral edema. Any significant hyperglycemia should be reported to receiving providers so that appropriate hospital interventions can be instituted.

EMS LEVELS OF CARE AND HOSPITAL NOTIFICATION

Determining the appropriate level of prehospital care dispatched to patients with stroke should take into consideration both the acuity of the patients' condition as well as the proximity of the closest available unit to rapidly expedite transport. Early studies did not show an effect on the admission rate, mortality rate, or disposition based on the level of transport for patients with stroke.[52] Although current ASA guidelines for EMS care of patients with stroke recommend dispatching the highest level of EMS care for these patients, it is important to recognize that for some EMS systems, it may be necessary to dispatch the closest available unit regardless of the level of care in cases when rapid transport to definitive care makes more sense than potentially timely on-scene management. Advanced life support (ALS) level of care may be better suited for the management of patients with acute stroke because of the need for paramedic-level intervention. ALS interventions may be required in as much as 29% of patients with stroke.[26] Despite patients transported by basic life support (BLS) arriving to the hospital sooner than ALS-transported patients, ALS patients were more likely to be seen sooner by an emergency physician on ED arrival. Ideally, patients with stroke should receive the highest level of prehospital care available, especially when there is an immediate need for critical intervention. However, this must be balanced with the immediate availability of other units, albeit of lower care levels, that may be able to initiate BLS stabilization and prompt transport to definitive care. This point is especially true for 2-tiered EMS systems using both BLS and ALS transport capabilities.

Early EMS communication and coordination with receiving hospitals has become a critical component to reducing delays to definitive care for patients with stroke. There is no doubt that stroke is considered a time-sensitive disease in which poor outcomes are directly related to increased time to fibrinolytic therapy.[44] Results from the most recent European Cooperate Acute Stroke Study, a double-blind,

STROKE ALERT/MEND* EXAM PREHOSPITAL CHECKLIST
MIAMI EMERGENCY NEUROLOGIC DEFICIT

DATE & TIMES					
Date:	Dispatch Time:	EMS Arrival Time:	EMS Departure Time:		ED Arrival Time:

BASIC DATA					
Patient Name			Age		Gender
Witness Name			Witness Phone		
Chief Complaint			BP	L /	R /
Last Time w/o Sxs		Glucose	Pulse		Resp

HISTORY	YES	NO
Severe Headache		
Head Trauma at Onset		

EXAMINATION	PERFORM ON SCENE	✓ IF ABNORMAL
Subarachnoid Hemorrhage?	Level of Consciousness (AVPU)	
	Neck Stiffness (cannot touch chin to chest)	
Cincinnati Prehospital Stroke Scale	Speech (repeat "You can't teach an old dog new tricks")	
	Facial Droop (show teeth or smile)	
	Arm Drift (close eyes and hold out both arms)	

STROKE ALERT CRITERIA	YES	NO
Time of onset < 6 hours?		
Any abnormal finding on examination?		
Deficit not likely due to head trauma?		
Blood glucose > 50? (if fingerstick possible)		

★★★ TRANSPORT **ALL** PATIENTS TO NEAREST APPROPRIATE "HOSPITAL"★★★
IF **YES** TO **ALL** STROKE ALERT CRITERIA, CALL **STROKE ALERT**, TRANSPORT PATIENT **URGENTLY**

DESTINATION HOSPITAL		HOSPITAL CONTACT	

PAST HISTORY / MEDICATIONS / ALLERGIES		
Past History	Recent → Surgery☐ Trauma☐ MI☐	**Medications**
Other:		
		Allergies

MEND EXAM	PERFORM EN ROUTE IF TIME ALLOWS	✓ IF ABNORMAL	
MENTAL STATUS	Level of Consciousness (AVPU)		
	Speech (repeat "You can't teach an old dog new tricks')		
	Questions (age, month)		
	Commands (close, open eyes)		
CRANIAL NERVES	Facial Droop (show teeth or smile)	R	L
	Visual Fields (four quadrants)	R	L
	Horizontal Gaze (side to side)	R	L
LIMBS	Motor—Arm Drift (close eyes and hold out both arms)	R	L
	Motor—Leg Drift (open eyes and lift each leg separately)	R	L
	Sensory—Arm and Leg (close eyes and touch, pinch)	R	L
	Coordination—Arm and Leg (finger to nose, heel to shin)	R	L

MANAGEMENT REMINDERS		
Do **NOT** treat hypertension	Do **NOT** allow aspiration → keep NPO, head up, O_2 2-4L	Do **NOT** give glucose → unless glucose < 50

STROKE-SPECIFIC REPORT TO EMERGENCY DEPARTMENT			
BASIC DATA	**SYMPTOM ONSET**	**SUPPLEMENTAL INFO**	**NEUROLOGIC EXAM**
• Age	• Last time w/o Sxs	• Recent surgery, trauma, MI	• Consci ousness
• Gender	• Hea d trauma	• Medic ations, Allergies	• Speech / language
• Chief Complaint	• Severe headache	• BP, Glucose	• Visua l fields
	• Seizure—staring or shaking	• Witness name, contact info	• Motor strength

© 2010, University of Miami Miller School of Medicine, Gordon Center for Research in Medical Education

Fig. 1. PHN checklist from the University of Miami Miller School of Medicine, Gordon Center for Research in Medical Education. (© 2010, University of Miami Miller School of Medicine, Gordon Center for Research in Medical Education.)

EMS RECEIVING HOSPITAL CONSIDERATIONS

Once arriving on scene and confirming the presence of a suspected acute stroke, the EMS provider should work to minimize scene time and provide rapid transport to definitive care; however, determining which is the most appropriate receiving facility requires a more complex algorithm than merely expediting scene and transport times. The nearest facility may not in fact be the most appropriate; there are several factors for consideration. Is the EMS system in a rural or resource-poor area, where total run times or transport times may exceed 60 to 90 minutes? Does the closest facility have 24-hour CT scan capabilities? Can the target facility provide t-PA, and if so, is the hospital also a certified stroke center? This last question merits particular consideration because studies continue to demonstrate decreased mortality and improved functional outcomes for patients treated at designated stroke centers.[61,62] In fact, it is now often recommended that EMS transport patients with acute stroke to the nearest *primary stroke center* (PSC) and not to the nearest facility unless patients require emergent intervention for conditions, such as cardiac arrest or airway management, in the case of BLS transport.[44] An example of a stroke disposition algorithm is shown in **Fig. 2**.

The most recent criteria for primary stroke centers are outlined in the 2011 Recommendations for the Establishment of Primary Stroke Centers (**Box 6**) as put forth by the Brain Attack Coalition.[63] In keeping with these recommendations, the NINDS 2012

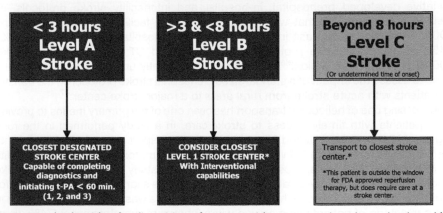

Fig. 2. Sample algorithm for disposition of patients with a suspected stroke as developed by the Golden Crescent Regional Advisory Council. (*Adapted from* Southeast Texas Regional Advisory Council (SETRAC). Houston, TX. Prehospital transport guidelines. Available at: http://www.setrac.org/Files/Committees/Trauma/SETRAC%20Transport%20Guidelines.pdf.)

Box 6
Criteria for designation of a primary stroke center

NINDS 2012 summary recommendations for the designation of PSCs

- Acute stroke team (class I, level A)
- Written protocols for stroke management (class I, level A)
- Integrated role for EMS (class I, level A)
- Timely laboratory testing and electrocardiogram completion (class I, level A)
- Quality assurance/Quality improvement resources (class I, level A)
- Establishment/use/availability of telemedicine (class I, level A)
- Available neurosurgery services (class I, level A)
- Timely CT/magnetic resonance imaging (MRI) *and interpretation* (class I, level A)
- Dedicated stroke unit (class I, level A) with telemetry capabilities (class I, level B)
- EMS should bypass closest facility to get to nearest PSC (class I, level B)
- EMS and transferring facilities should consider helicopter transport to reduce transport times (class II, level B)
- MRI for admitted patients (class I, level A) and Computed tomography angiogram/Magnetic resonance angiography capabilities (class I, level B)
- Transthoracic echocardiogram, transesophageal echocardiography, (class I, level A), or cardiac MRI capabilities (class IIb, level C)

---

update noted that greater than half of the US population now lives in a state or county in which patients are preferentially diverted to PSCs for acute stroke care.[64] For populations that do not have prompt access to a PSC, there are notable disparities in the quality of stroke care, which is most evident when comparing urban and rural areas.[65] Emerging data suggests that this gap can be reduced through the targeted development of regional stroke networks and aggressive provider education plans. As an example of how such plans can be designed and implemented, the Montana Stroke Initiative developed prehospital, in-hospital, and interfacility stroke protocols, as well as a stroke toolkit that was provided to remote facilities. Between 2004 and 2008, there was an increase in the availability of prehospital screening tools (49%–74%), written ED stroke protocols (58%–85%), and CT scan availability (67%–100%) in this remote region.[66] A similar trial is currently underway in Australia and aims to assess the impact of a standardized prehospital stroke protocol on the transfer of patients with acute stroke from rural areas to a major stroke center.[67]

Increasing use of helicopter transport has been one of the primary means to provide rural patients with timely access to stroke care. In a study performed in the rural regions of Southeastern United States, air medical transport allowed 65 of 85 patients with stroke to arrive to an ED within 135 minutes of symptom onset.[68] Such benefits were also found in a large, prospective, observational study from the Austrian Stroke Registry in which the highest rates of fibrinolysis and the shortest arrival times were for those patients transported by helicopter services. There was a substantial increase in the percentage of patients who arrived within 2 hours of symptom onset (74% direct via air transport, 52% direct via ambulance transport), and patients transported directly from the field to a stroke center by helicopter had t-PA rates of 24.0% compared with ambulance transport alone (8.7%).[69] When considering air medical transport, however, it is important to remember that air transport is only significantly faster if the transport distance is greater than 10 miles from hospital.[70]

If helicopter services are unavailable (eg, because of poor weather conditions), telemedicine is an evolving means to provide high-level stroke care. Remote consultation with PSCs through telemedicine was another modality trialed in the Montana Stroke Initiative[63]; this service is also finding validity in other regions. In Georgia, infrastructure has been developed to provide rural EDs with access to neurologic consultation from a remote PSC, 24 hours a day, 7 days a week.[71] Consultation services included real-time radiologist interpretation of head CTs, NIHSS evaluation by a neurologist, and recommendations for t-PA administration. Within the first year of implementation, 12 patients in this system had received t-PA out of a total of 75 evaluated patients with stroke. In a rural catchment area that was previously unable to provide thrombolytic therapy at all, the average door-to-needle time was 105 minutes. Although not a substitute for in-house neurologic services or for ongoing poststroke care, telemedicine is providing access to early interventional therapies that would otherwise be unavailable to remote populations.

SUMMARY

Significant advances have been made in the prehospital care of patients with stroke over the past decade. Although the earlier discoveries of fibrinolytic therapy had been in the forefront of acute stroke care, it is becoming more apparent that an important factor in stroke outcomes is highly dependent on the timing of medication administration. The therapeutic window of t-PA administration has increased from 3.0 to 4.5 hours, but the fact remains that no matter the window, the sooner fibrinolytic therapy can be instituted the better. Recent research supports the concept that the prehospital phase of acute stroke care can improve this door-to-needle time. Improving systems, such as early dispatch and notification to EMS crews of a possible stroke through better education of the public as well as dispatcher recognition of stroke, improving EMS-provider identification, and reducing scene time to focused care and rapid transport to an appropriate receiving facility, help reduce that door-to-needle time. Early EMS notification to receiving hospitals has been shown to reduce significant time intervals and to reduce the delay to definitive therapy. Such a Hawthorne effect has a downstream impact, allowing receiving hospitals to be more prepared for possible patients with stroke. Similar to the current approaches to other time-sensitive diseases, such as trauma and myocardial infarction, understanding the EMS system and factors within both the public understanding and EMS response is integral to making positive changes in how patients with acute stroke are managed.

REFERENCES

1. The National Institute of Neurological Disorders and Stroke rt-PA Stroke Study Group. Tissue plasminogen activator for acute ischemic stroke. N Engl J Med 1995;333:1581–7.
2. Hacke W, Kaste M, Bluhmki E, et al. Thrombolysis with alteplase 3 to 4.5 hours after acute ischemic stroke. N Engl J Med 2008;359:1317–29.
3. del Zoppo G, Saver J, Jauch E, et al. Expansion of the time window for treatment of acute ischemic stroke patients with intravenous tissue plasminogen activator: a science advisory from the American Heart Association/American Stroke Association. Stroke 2009;40:2945–8.
4. Carpenter C, Kein S, Milne W, et al. Thrombolytic therapy for acute ischemic stroke beyond three hours. J Emerg Med 2011;40:82–92.

5. Thom T, Haase N, Rosamond W, et al. Heart disease and stroke statistics – 2006 update: a report from the American Heart Association Statistics Committee and Stroke Statistics Subcommittee. Circulation 2006;113:e85–151.
6. Centers for Disease Control and Prevention. Prehospital and hospital delays after stroke onset – United States 2005-2006. MMWR Morb Mortal Wkly Rep 2007;18: 474–8.
7. Pepe P, Zachariah B, Sayre M, et al. Ensuring the chain of recovery for stroke in your community. Acad Emerg Med 1998;5:352–8.
8. National Institute of Neurological Disorders and Stroke Symposium. Improving the stroke chain of recovery for acute stroke in your community. Task Force Reports. December 12–13, 2002. Available at: http://www.ninds.nih.gov/news_ and_events/proceedings/stroke_2002/acute_stroke_choosing.htm.   Accessed electronically on January 19, 2012.
9. Suyama J, Crocco T. Prehospital care of the stroke patient. Emerg Med Clin North Am 2002;20:537–52.
10. Wester P, Radberg J, Lundgren B, et al. Factors associated with delayed admission and in-hospital delays in acute stroke and TIA, a prospective multicenter study. Stroke 1999;30:40–8.
11. Davis S. Strengthening the link: the critical role of children in the stroke chain of recovery. Stroke 2008;39:2695–6.
12. Rossnagel K, Jan Jungehulsing G, Nolte C, et al. Out-of-hospital delays in patients with acute stroke. Ann Emerg Med 2004;44:476–83.
13. Kothari R, Jauch E, Broderick J, et al. Acute stroke: delay to presentation and emergency department evaluation. Ann Emerg Med 1999;33:3–8.
14. Keskin O, Kalemoglu M, Ulusoy R. A clinic investigation into prehospital and emergency department delays in acute stroke care. Med Princ Pract 2005;14: 408–12.
15. Schroeder E, Rosamond W, Morris D, et al. Determinants of use of emergency medical services in a population with stroke symptoms, the second delay in accessing stroke healthcare (DASH II) study. Stroke 2000;31:2591–6.
16. Mikulik R, Bunt L, Hrdlicka D, et al. Calling 911 in response to stroke: a nationwide study assessing definitive individual behavior. Stroke 2008;39:1844–9.
17. Mikulik R, Goldemund D, Reif M, et al. Calling 911 in response to stroke: no change following a four-year educational campaign. Cerebrovasc Dis 2011;32: 342–8.
18. Marx JJ, Nedelmann M, Haertle B, et al. An educational multimedia campaign has differential effects on public stroke knowledge and care-seeking behavior. J Neurol 2008;255:378–84.
19. Muller-Nordhorn J, Nolte C, Rossnagel K, et al. Knowledge about risk factors for stroke: a population-based survey with 28,090 participants. Stroke 2006;37: 946–50.
20. Kleindorfer D, Lindsell C, Moomaw C, et al. Which stroke symptoms prompt a 911 call? A population-based study. Am J Emerg Med 2010;28:607–12.
21. Adeoye O, Lindsell C, Broderick J, et al. Emergency medical services use by stroke patients: a population-based study. Am J Emerg Med 2009;27:141–5.
22. Roebers S, Wagner M, Ritter M, et al. Attitudes and current practice of primary care physicians in acute stroke management. Stroke 2007;38:1298–303.
23. Rosamond W, Gorton R, Hinn A, et al. Rapid response to stroke symptoms: the delay in accessing stroke healthcare (DASH) study. Acad Emerg Med 1998;5:45–51.
24. Williams O, Noble J. 'Hip hop stroke' – a stroke educational program for elementary school children living in high-risk community. Stroke 2008;39:2809–16.

25. Hurwitz A, Brice J, Overby B, et al. Directed use of the Cincinnati Prehospital Stroke Scale by laypersons. Prehosp Emerg Care 2005;9:292–6.
26. Kothari R, Barsan W, Brott T, et al. Frequency and accuracy of prehospital diagnosis of acute stroke. Stroke 1995;26:937–41.
27. Ellison S, Gratton M, Schwab R, et al. Prehospital dispatch assessment of stroke. Mo Med 2004;101:64–6.
28. Rosamond W, Evenson K, Schroeder E, et al. Calling emergency medical services for acute stroke: a study of 9-1-1 tapes. Prehosp Emerg Care 2005;9: 19–23.
29. Buck B, Starkman S, Eckstein M, et al. Dispatcher recognition of stroke using the national academy medical priority dispatch system. Stroke 2009;40:2027–30.
30. Ramanujam P, Castillo E, Patel E, et al. Prehospital transport time intervals for acute stroke patients. J Emerg Med 2009;37:40–5.
31. Govindarajan P, Ghilarducci D, McCulloch C, et al. Comparative evaluation of stroke triage algorithms for emergency medical dispatchers (MeDS): prospective cohort study protocol. BMC Neurol 2011;27:14.
32. Crocco T, Kothari R, Sayre M, et al. A nationwide prehospital stroke survey. Prehosp Emerg Care 1999;3:201–6.
33. Hourihane J, Clark W. Clinical assessment and outcome scales in acute stroke. Neuroimaging Clin N Am 1999;9:539–52.
34. Tirshwell D, Longstreth W, Becker K, et al. Shortening the NIH stroke scale for use in the prehospital setting. Stroke 2002;33:2801–6.
35. Kothari R, Hall K, Brott T, et al. Early stroke recognition: developing an out-of-hospital NIH stroke scale. Acad Emerg Med 1997;4:986–90.
36. Kothari R, Pancioli A, Liu T, et al. Cincinnati prehospital stroke scale: reproducibility and validity. Ann Emerg Med 1999;33:373–8.
37. Frendl D, Strauss D, Underhill B, et al. Lack of impact of paramedic training and use of the Cincinnati prehospital stroke scale patient identification and on-scene time. Stroke 2009;40:754–6.
38. Kidwell C, Saver J, Schubert G, et al. Design and prospective analysis of the Los Angeles Prehospital Stroke Screen (LAPSS). Prehosp Emerg Care 1998;2:267–73.
39. Kidwell C, Starkman S, Eckstein M, et al. Identifying stroke in the field: prospective validation of the Los Angeles Prehospital Stroke Screen (LAPSS). Stroke 2000;31:71–6.
40. Llanes J, Kidwell C, Starkman S, et al. The Los Angeles Motor Scale (LAMS): a new measure to characterize stroke severity in the field. Prehosp Emerg Care 2004;8:46–50.
41. Bray J, Martin J, Cooper G, et al. Paramedic identification of stroke: community validation of the Melbourne Ambulance Stroke Screen. Cerebrovasc Dis 2005; 20:28–33.
42. Bray J, Coughlan K, Barger B, et al. Paramedic diagnosis of stroke: examining long-term use of the Melbourne Ambulance Stroke Screen (MASS) in the field. Stroke 2010;41:1363–6.
43. Fisher M, Ginsberg M. Current concepts of the ischemic penumbra. Stroke 2004; 35:2657–8.
44. Adams H, Del Zoppo G, Alberts M, et al. Guidelines for the early management of patients with acute ischemic stroke. Circulation 2007;115:e478–534.
45. Leonardi-Bee J, Bath P, Phillips S, et al. Blood pressure and clinical outcomes in the International Stroke Trial. Stroke 2002;33:1315–20.
46. Phillips S. Pathophysiology and management of hypertension in acute ischemic stroke. Hypertension 1994;23:131–6.

Evaluation of CVT is similar to other types of stroke, and includes basic blood work with coagulation studies, as well as an initial noncontrast head CT and neurology consult. As in other types of ischemic stroke, the first noncontrast head CT can be negative, and studies have shown an approximate sensitivity for CVT of only 30%.[14] Noncontrast CT findings include hyperdensity of the dural veins or the dense delta sign. The classic empty delta sign, which is due to lack of flow, can be seen on a venous contrast-enhanced CT, which is the next step if clinical suspicion is high, and the noncontrast CT is normal.

Anticoagulation remains the cornerstone of CVT treatment. This can be achieved via unfractionated heparin or weight-based low molecular weight heparin (class 2a, level B).[14] Treatment of secondary problems such as associated infection (eg, meningitis, abscess), increased intracranial pressure (ICP), and seizure should also be initiated. Antibiotics are indicated if infection is suspected. If there are signs of increased ICP, patients should undergo appropriate treatments, including acetazolamide, shunts or other decompression interventions with the aid of neurosurgical consultants. While antiepileptics are indicated if the patient has had a seizure, there is no evidence that these patients need to be loaded with antiepileptics as prophylaxis (class 3, level C).[14]

EVALUATION

The initial evaluation of patients with suspected acute ischemic stroke must be swift to facilitate treatment within accepted timelines.[2,16] The Stroke Chain of Survival guidelines are published by the AHA/ASA to promote prompt recognition and treatment of acute ischemic stroke. The guidelines emphasize the seven Ds: (1) detection (of symptoms), (2) dispatch (of emergency medical services [EMS] to the patient), (3) delivery (of the patient to the emergency department), (4) door (noting time of arrival), (5) data (gathering history, physical examination, laboratory tests, and CT scan), (6) decision (does the patient qualify for treatment), and (7) drug (administration of thrombolytic).[17]

The AHA/ASA have also published Get With the Guidelines recommendations in hopes of further improving the management of stroke. These guidelines were updated in 2010 and provide important timeline goals (**Fig. 3**). The first 10 minutes comprise the initial evaluation, including completing a history and neurologic examination with National Institutes of Health (NIH) stroke scale score, ordering the CT scan, obtaining intravenous access and laboratory tests, and calling a neurologist for a stroke consultation, where possible. Within 25 minutes, the patient should have completed a noncontrast head CT. This should be read by a qualified radiologist within 45 minutes, and thrombolytics should be administered within one hour of presentation.

The assessment and treatment of a stroke patient can be managed in many emergency departments with advanced planning. However, this streamlined process is facilitated at designated stroke centers,[18] which have rapid response protocols, integrated systems, and increased experience in completing an efficient evaluation of the possible stroke patient. History and physical examination provide the basis for diagnosis of acute stroke. CT scan is usually normal or age-appropriate in acute ischemic stroke, and is used to exclude other diagnoses that may preclude intervention. Careful attention must be paid to the many stroke mimics. The decision to treat must consider important contraindications to fibrinolytics. For these reasons, physicians at stroke centers are often more comfortable administering thrombolytics than the average community emergency medicine physician. Moreover, comprehensive stroke centers also have the ability to do endovascular interventions for patients who fall outside of thrombolytic guidelines.

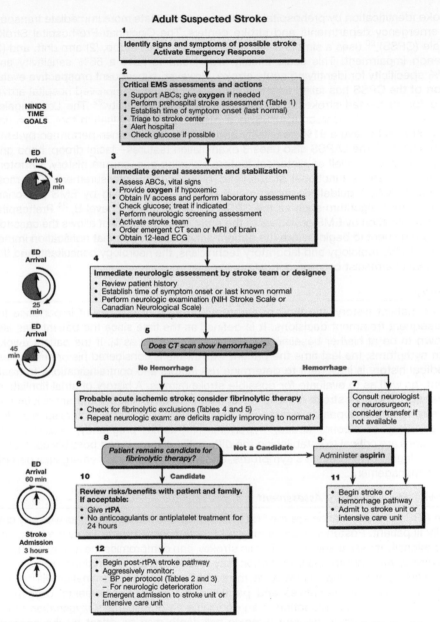

Adult Suspected Stroke

1
Identify signs and symptoms of possible stroke
Activate Emergency Response

2
Critical EMS assessments and actions
- Support ABCs; give **oxygen** if needed
- Perform prehospital stroke assessment (Table 1)
- Establish time of symptom onset (last normal)
- Triage to stroke center
- Alert hospital
- Check glucose if possible

NINDS
TIME
GOALS

ED
Arrival
10 min

3
Immediate general assessment and stabilization
- Assess ABCs, vital signs
- Provide **oxygen** if hypoxemic
- Obtain IV access and perform laboratory assessments
- Check glucose; treat if indicated
- Perform neurologic screening assessment
- Activate stroke team
- Order emergent CT scan or MRI of brain
- Obtain 12-lead ECG

ED
Arrival
25 min

4
Immediate neurologic assessment by stroke team or designee
- Review patient history
- Establish time of symptom onset or last known normal
- Perform neurologic examination (NIH Stroke Scale or Canadian Neurological Scale)

ED
Arrival
45 min

5
Does CT scan show hemorrhage?

No Hemorrhage   Hemorrhage

6
Probable acute ischemic stroke; consider fibrinolytic therapy
- Check for fibrinolytic exclusions (Tables 4 and 5)
- Repeat neurologic exam: are deficits rapidly improving to normal?

7
Consult neurologist or neurosurgeon; consider transfer if not available

8
Patient remains candidate for fibrinolytic therapy?   Not a Candidate

9
Administer **aspirin**

ED
Arrival
60 min

10   Candidate
Review risks/benefits with patient and family. If acceptable:
- Give rtPA
- No anticoagulants or antiplatelet treatment for 24 hours

11
- Begin stroke or hemorrhage pathway
- Admit to stroke unit or intensive care unit

Stroke
Admission
3 hours

12
- Begin post-rtPA stroke pathway
- Aggressively monitor:
  – BP per protocol (Tables 2 and 3)
  – For neurologic deterioration
- Emergent admission to stroke unit or intensive care unit

Fig. 3. Goals for management of patients with suspected stroke. (*From* Jauch EC, Cucchiara B, Adeoye O, et al. Part 11: adult stroke: 2010 American Heart Association Guidelines for Cardiopulmonary Resuscitation and Emergency Cardiovascular Care. Circulation 2010;122 [18 Suppl 3]:S818–28; with permission.)

Prehospital Evaluation

Appropriate prehospital evaluation of the stroke patient and notification of the receiving facility are beneficial for adherence to the strict interventional timelines.[19] Several prehospital EMS scales have been proposed to improve the accuracy of stroke identification by prehospital providers, and facilitate more immediate transport to emergency departments and stroke centers. The Cincinnati Pre-hospital Stroke Scale (CPSS),[20] uses a simple 3-tier evaluation: (1) facial droop, (2) arm drift, and (3) speech impairment. This scale initially was found to have a 66% sensitivity and 87% specificity for identifying acute stroke. However, subsequent prospective evaluation of the CPSS has failed to show increased capture or improved hospital arrival time for suspected strokes[21] as well as only 42% sensitivity.[22] The Los Angeles Pre-hospital Stroke Screen (LAPSS) is a more extensive evaluation tool, which has been shown to have a 91% sensitivity and 97% specificity when performed by EMS technicians.[23] The LAPSS also uses 3 examination features—facial droop, hand grip and arm drift—as well as historical factors including age, seizure history, symptom duration, baseline functional status, and blood glucose measurement. The most recent AHA/ASA guidelines recommend prehospital screening by EMS personnel with a stroke algorithm such as the CPSS or LAPSS (class 1, level B).[24] Prehospital radio notification by EMS providers to the emergency department allows the cascade of management to begin before the patient arrives. Conveying that notification immediately to the radiology and laboratory technicians, the neurology consultant, and the hospital pharmacist can prevent delays in care.

History

In the patient history, the time of symptom onset is of paramount importance for subsequent treatment decisions. It is defined as the time since the patient was last known to be at his/her baseline state and is recognized as t_0. If the patient awoke with symptoms, the last time the patient was awake is considered his or her t_0. Past medical history is important to determine risk factors and contraindications to treatment, as well as to evaluate for possible stroke mimics. A history of atrial fibrillation, older age, and prior stroke or transient ischemic attack (TIA) are important risk factors for stroke, and all appear to increase poststroke mortality.[25] Other factors such as diabetes, drug or alcohol abuse, hypertension, trauma, pregnancy, seizures, and migraines are critical to establishing the differential diagnosis and possible confounding etiologies of the patient's symptoms, and will help guide early emergency department management.

Airway and Circulatory Assessment

The ABCs of resuscitation are the first priority in stroke management, as with any critically ill patient. Posterior circulation and brainstem ischemic stroke syndromes, and occasionally massive anterior ischemic strokes, can compromise the airway. Securing the airway with endotracheal intubation may be required. Consideration must be made in the timing of securing an airway, as the patient's neurologic examination will be difficult to assess after sedatives and paralytics are given. Supplemental oxygen for patients not requiring intubation is an ongoing area of research. Oxygenation of the ischemic penumbra to prevent hypoxic cell death may be offset by the negative effects produced by free oxygen radicals. At this time, there does not appear to be a role for supplemental oxygen in nonhypoxic ischemic stroke patients,[26] and oxygen is only recommended to maintain a saturation of greater than 92%.[24] However, there is interest in revisiting this area in patients treated with thrombolytics.

Circulatory assessment includes careful monitoring and management of blood pressure. Many stroke patients have a past medical history of high blood pressure, which may change their cerebral perfusion oxygenation curve. Acute blood pressure elevations seen in early stroke may be compensatory as the body tries to provide increased cerebral perfusion pressure to overcome tissue ischemia. There is likely also an acute stress response, causing a catecholamine surge and resultant elevation in blood pressure. This elevated blood pressure can cause an ischemic stroke to convert to an intracranial hemorrhage at the site of the damaged tissue, particularly in the setting of thrombolytics. Therefore, a balance must be maintained between the competing risks of bleeding or worsening the ischemic penumbra.

Multiple studies[27–30] have shown an increase in poor outcomes in stroke patients with hypotension, as well as severe hypertension. However, there is little scientific evidence that acutely lowering blood pressure leads to improved outcomes. A recent randomized, placebo-controlled trial looking at the effect of lowering blood pressure in ischemic stroke patients with candesartan versus placebo[31] failed to show improved outcomes with lowered pressures in the treatment group, and in fact, showed harm. Conversely, retrospective reviews[32] have found a positive correlation between baseline systolic blood pressure and size of post-tPA hemorrhage hematoma size.

Permissive hypertension is recommended in most acute ischemic stroke patients. Achieving a blood pressure that allows administration of thrombolytics is the goal in the appropriate candidate (blood pressure <185/110 mm HG). A patient who is otherwise a tPA candidate presenting with a blood pressure >185/110 mm Hg can be given labetalol, nitropaste, or a nicardipine infusion (**Box 1**).[24] These treatment guidelines from 2007 are based on expert consensus and limited data, and the target goals have not been rigorously studied. With new data emerging regarding possible harm in acutely lowering blood pressure in acute ischemic stroke,[31] as well as the lack of documented benefit, aggressive blood pressure control continues to be discouraged. Only hypertensive patients who are tPA candidates, or those with severely elevated blood pressures (systolic blood pressure >220 mm Hg and/or diastolic blood pressure >120 mm Hg) should receive antihypertensives (class 1, level C).[24]

Temperature and Glucose Control

Temperature and a fingerstick blood glucose level are important vital signs for presumed stroke patients. Sepsis and hypoglycemia are routine mimics of stroke symptoms. In no case should thrombolytics be given without this crucial information. Ischemic stroke patients presenting with fever have increased mortality,[24] but treating fever has not been shown to improve outcomes.[33] A thorough search for an underlying cause should be undertaken, and any findings should be treated concurrently with stroke management. Therapeutic hypothermia, widely used as neuroprotective therapy for cardiac arrest patients, is a current area of research in ischemic stroke. There have been some small trials showing a modest benefit in stroke patients, but large trials, and trials including tPA patients, are lacking.[34]

Poststroke hyperglycemia is common and can be a result of stress, underlying diabetes mellitus, or other medical conditions. Recent literature comparing initial serum blood glucose levels in stroke patients to outcomes at 3 months, measured by modified Rankin score (mRS) (**Table 1**), found a sharp decline in favorable outcomes with levels below 66 mg/dL or above 130 mg/dL.[35] A meta-analysis of the topic found that nondiabetic patients with an admission serum glucose greater than 110 to 126 mg/dL had an increased risk of in-hospital or 30-day mortality.[36] They also found that nondiabetic survivors of stroke with hyperglycemia on admission had poorer functional outcomes. There was no similar association found in diabetic patients. Similarly, a recent prospective observational study looking at a thrombolysis stroke registry found admission hyperglycemia to be an independent predictor of poor outcome (mRS >2), as well as an increased risk of symptomatic intracerebral hemorrhage (odds ratio [OR] 2.86, $P<.001$).[37] This significance was seen at serum glucose levels greater than 120 mg/dL for poor outcomes and at greater than 180 mg/dL for hemorrhage. Data analyzed

Box 1
Approach to arterial hypertension in acute ischemic stroke

Indication that patient is eligible for treatment with intravenous rtPA or other acute reperfusion intervention

Blood pressure level

Systolic blood pressure >185 mm Hg or diastolic blood pressure >110 mm Hg

Labetalol 10–20 mg intravenously over 1–2 minutes, may repeat ×1; or Nitropaste 1–2 inches; or Nicardipine infusion, 5 mg/h, titrate up by 2.5 mg/h at 5- to 15-min intervals, maximum dose 15 mg/h; when desired blood pressure attained, reduce to 3 mg/h

If blood pressure does not decline and remains >185/110 mm Hg, do not administer rtPA

Management of blood pressure during and after treatment with rtPA or other acute reperfusion intervention

Monitor blood pressure every 15 minutes during treatment and then for another 2 hours, then every 30 minutes for 6 hours, and then every hour for 16 hours

Blood pressure level

Systolic blood pressure 180–230 mm Hg or diastolic blood pressure 105–120 mm Hg

Labetalol 10 mg intravenously over 1–2 minutes, may repeat every 10–20 minutes, maximum dose of 300 mg; or labetalol 10 mg intravenously followed by an infusion at 2–8 mg/min

Systolic blood pressure >230 mm Hg or diastolic blood pressure 121–140 mm Hg

Labetalol 10 mg intravenously over 1–2 minutes, may repeat every 10–20 minutes, maximum dose of 300 mg; or labetalol 10 mg intravenously followed by an infusion at 2–8 mg/min; or nicardipine infusion, 5 mg/h, titrate up to desired effect by increasing 2.5 mg/h every 5 minutes to maximum of 15 mg/h

If blood pressure not controlled, consider sodium nitroprusside

From Adams HP Jr, del Zoppo G, Alberts MJ, et al. Guidelines for the early management of adults with ischemic stroke: a guideline from the American Heart Association/American Stroke Association Stroke Council, Clinical Cardiology Council, Cardiovascular Radiology and Intervention Council, and the Atherosclerotic Peripheral Vascular Disease and Quality of Care Outcomes in Research Interdisciplinary Working Groups: the American Academy of Neurology affirms the value of this guideline as an educational tool for neurologists. Stroke 2007;38(5): 1655–711; with permission.

Table 1
Modified Rankin scale

Score	Description
0	No symptoms at all
1	No significant disability despite symptoms; able to carry out all usual duties and activities
2	Slight disability; unable to carry out all previous activities, but able to look after own affairs without assistance
3	Moderate disability; requiring some help, but able to walk without assistance
4	Moderately severe disability; unable to walk without assistance and unable to attend to own bodily needs without assistance
5	Severe disability; bedridden, incontinent and requiring constant nursing care and attention
6	Dead

from the NINDS trial also found an increased risk of hemorrhage in patients with hyper-glycemia (OR 1.75/100 mg/dL increase in admission glucose, P = .02).[38] Given the clear evidence of hyperglycemia associated poor outcomes, the AHA/ASA guidelines give a class 2 recommendation for the treatment of hyperglycemia and give a value of greater than 140 to 185 mg/dL as an initial treatment starting point.

Physical Examination

The variety of stroke presentations and subjectivity of portions of the physical exam-ination can make diagnosing stroke difficult.[39] Coma, loss of consciousness, neck stiffness, seizures, headache, vomiting, or a diastolic blood pressure of greater than 110 mm Hg increase the likelihood of hemorrhagic stroke.[40] The National Institutes of Health Stroke Scale (NIHSS) (**Box 2**) is an 11-item score set that is designed to be used by every level of health care provider, and allows emergency physicians and neurologists across the country to standardize neurologic assessments with high inter-rater reliability.[41] It provides a quantitative value for the baseline neurologic examination that can then be repeated throughout the patient's hospital course.

The NIHSS is scored from zero to 42, with less than 5 indicating a minor stroke, and greater than 20 to 25 a severe stroke. It should be noted, however, that a score of zero does not preclude stroke,[42] and posterior circulation strokes in particular can be missed. Abnormal gait was the most common sign found in patients with an NIHSS score of zero and magnetic resonance imaging (MRI) evidence of stroke. Headache, vertigo, and nausea were the most common symptoms in these patients. The scale also seems to favor identification of left hemispheric injury and often underestimates right-sided infarcts.[43] This scale has important implications for management,[2,16] and should be performed quickly by the emergency physician or consulting neurologist upon the patient's arrival. The NIHSS carries a class 1, level B evidence rating by the AHA/ASA, and all emergency physicians should be familiar with this scale. NIHSS pocket cards are available, and it is recommended that the scale be practiced on a variety of patients to ensure practitioner familiarity with implementation. The decision regarding whether to administer thrombolytics is in part guided by a patient's score on the NIHSS.

Laboratory Data

To expedite management, laboratory tests, including serum electrolytes, renal function tests, a complete blood cell count including platelets, coagulation studies, and markers of cardiac ischemia[24] should be collected and sent to the laboratory prior to imaging. The tests can be run and interpreted during imaging. An EKG should be performed on all stroke patients, but obtaining the EKG should not delay neuroimaging. These tests further identify stroke mimics, and may provide data that could exclude a patient from treatment or highlight other concerns. A low albumin and hemoglobin concentra-tion and a high creatinine on arrival are associated with higher mortality.[25] The effects of hyperglycemia have been discussed previously in this article.

The results of platelet and coagulopathic studies may be of interest, also. Although large trials are lacking, Rost and colleagues,[44] in a retrospective study, found that unsuspected coagulopathy (international normalized ratio [INR]$\geq$1.7 or platelets less than or equal to 100,000/μL) was only found in 0.4% of patients. Cucchiara and colleagues,[45] in another retrospective review, found that only 0.3% of patients had unsuspected platelet counts of less than 100,000μL. Both of these studies suggest that unless a coagulopathy or thrombocytopenia is suspected due to prior illness or medications, it is rare to find. These studies also suggest that the benefits of thrombol-ysis may outweigh the risks of waiting on laboratory results given the infrequency of

---

Box 2
NIHSS score

1a. Level of consciousness	0 = Alert; keenly responsive
	1 = Not alert, but arousable by minor stimulation
	2 = Not alert; requires repeated stimulation
	3 = Unresponsive or responds only with reflex
1b. Level of consciousness questions:	0 = Both answers correct
What is the month?	1 = Answers 1 question correctly
What is your age?	2 = Answers 2 questions correctly
1c. Level of consciousness commands:	0 = Performs both tasks correctly
Open and close your eyes	1 = Performs 1 task correctly
Grip and release your hand	2 = Performs neither task correctly
2. Best gaze	0 = Normal
	1 = Partial gaze palsy
	2 = Forced deviation
3. Visual	0 = No visual loss
	1 = Partial hemianopia
	2 = Complete hemianopia
	3 = Bilateral hemianopia
4. Facial palsy	0 = Normal symmetric movements
	1 = Minor paralysis
	2 = Partial paralysis
	3 = Complete paralysis of one or both sides
5. Motor arm	0 = No drift
5a. Left arm	1 = Drift
5b. Right arm	2 = Some effort against gravity
	3 = No effort against gravity; limb falls
	4 = No movement
6. Motor leg	0 = No drift
6a. Left leg	1 = Drift
6b. Right leg	2 = Some effort against gravity
	3 = No effort against gravity
	4 = No movement
7. Limb ataxia	0 = Absent
	1 = Present in 1 limb
	2 = Present in 2 limbs
8. Sensory	0 = Normal; no sensory loss
	1 = Mild-to-moderate sensory loss
	2 = Severe to total sensory loss
9. Best language	0 = No aphasia; normal
	1 = Mild to moderate aphasia
	2 = Severe aphasia
	3 = Mute, global aphasia
10. Dysarthria	0 = Normal
	1 = Mild-to-moderate dysarthria
	2 = Severe dysarthria
11. Extinction and inattention	0 = No abnormality
	1 = Visual, tactile, auditory, spatial, or personal inattention
	2 = Profound hemi-inattention or extinction

Total score = 0–42.

Reprinted with permission of Elsevier.

abnormal values. A small study showed improved door-to-decision times (84 to 40 min, $P<.001$) when a point-of-care system was implemented for stroke blood tests, rather than waiting for central laboratory results.[46]

Imaging

There is a low overall sensitivity for the clinical examination in diagnosing stroke, but the likelihood of stroke does increase with certain findings, including facial droop, arm drift, or speech impairment (positive likelihood ratio [LR] = 5.5; 95% confidence interval [CI], 3.3–9.1).[39] Hemorrhagic versus ischemic stroke can often be differentiated clinically, but there can be overlap in the clinical findings. Appropriate neuroimaging should always be acquired to distinguish these vascular disturbances.

Imaging may accomplish three things. First, and most importantly, it can rule out hemorrhagic infarcts. Second, it may allow the clinician to identify the occluded vessel. Last, depending on the imaging modality and elapsed time from the onset of symptoms, it may identify the infarcted area as well as the surrounding ischemic penumbra. A noncontrast head CT scan is the initial imaging modality of choice. It should be performed within 25 minutes and interpreted within 45 minutes of the patient's arrival.[17] Meeting these time goals allows a hemorrhagic stroke to be ruled out with time remaining to consider, prepare, and administer fibrinolytics. These times are recommended in the 2010 AHA/ASA guidelines.

CT angiography (CTA) is the noninvasive gold standard imaging modality for locating occluded intracranial vessels. Modalities such as CT perfusion imaging have a higher specificity for ischemic stroke, but require a longer time to acquire and cause additional radiation exposure. CT perfusion is a qualitative assessment using a bolus of intravenous contrast to determine cerebral blood flow. The Xenon-enhanced CT can assess the cerebral blood flow quantitatively. Areas of infarct will have no blood flow, and the ischemic penumbra around the infarct will have decreased flow, illuminating potentially reversible areas of dysfunction.[47] The availability of this technology is limited, and its use remains investigational.

MRI has the advantage of isolating even smaller areas of ischemia. Additionally, it has a higher sensitivity, and in the right facility, can be used efficiently for the initial evaluation of acute ischemic stroke.[48–52] Diffusion-weighted MRI (DWI) can detect very early ischemic insults to within the first few minutes and can illustrate lesions in the posterior fossa where CT imaging falls short. Perfusion MRI is similar to perfusion CT in that it uses a bolus of contrast to identify areas of decreased cerebral blood flow. It can also give additional information regarding cerebral blood volume and mean transit time.[53] A multimodal approach to MRI includes DWI, perfusion-weighted, magnetic resonance angiography (MRA), gradient echo (GRE), and fluid-attenuated inversion recovery (FLAIR) sequences (further information on stroke imaging is available elsewhere in this issue). Limitations of MRI include higher cost, limited availability, and more time and patient cooperation than noncontrast CT scans. A review of the literature comparing CT to MRI indicates that more studies with larger numbers are needed before definitive conclusions regarding the optimal imaging regimen can be made.[54] At this time, noncontrast head CT is the only imaging required to make a decision regarding thrombolysis.

TREATMENT
Thrombolytics

Before FDA approval of thrombolytics for acute ischemic stroke, treatment was limited to care in a stroke unit and aspirin within 48 hours. In a select population of stroke sufferers, outcomes have improved with the addition of thrombolytic therapy. Thrombolytics cause the activation of plasminogen, which breaks down the fibrin-bound clot which is causing the ischemic insult. Recombinant tPA is the most fibrin-specific of these agents. It undergoes first-pass metabolism by the liver, which gives it a much shorter half-life (4–6 minutes) than other agents.[55,56] Previous research with streptokinase[57,58] found little benefit, and increased morbidity and mortality when used in acute ischemic stroke. Currently, tPA is the only approved thrombolytic in the United States. Since its approval, there have been many studies and discussions regarding the optimum use of this intervention.

The landmark trial published in 1995 by NINDS[2] resulted in the FDA's approval of tPA for treatment of stroke. This trial investigated the administration of tPA within three hours of stroke onset, and monitored outcomes at 24 hours and three months (**Table 2**). Improvement was measured by a change of four points on the NIHSS. No improvement was found with tPA therapy at 24 hours. The three-month results measured functionality using four outcome scales (modified Rankin, Glasgow, Barthel index and NIHSS). The study found that patients treated with tPA were at least 30% more likely to have minimal or no disability at three months as measured by all four outcome scales (Rankin 0–1, Glasgow 1, Barthel 95–100, NIHSS 0–1). There was an increase in symptomatic intracerebral hemorrhage in the tPA arm (6.4% in tPA versus 0.6% in placebo, $P<.001$), but there was no difference in mortality between the two groups.

A similar trial done around the same time found different results.[59] The European Cooperative Acute Stroke Study (ECASS I), the first of three ECASS studies, investigated the administration of tPA given within 6 hours of symptom onset for moderate-to-severe stroke. This study found some functional improvement in the tPA arm, but also found a higher mortality rate at 30 days. The authors concluded that tPA could not be universally recommended based on these results. However, this trial had a longer onset to treatment parameter (6 hours) and used a larger dose of tPA (1.1 mg/kg) than the NINDS trial. ECASS II,[60] published a few years after ECASS I, also found no benefit with administration of tPA within 6 hours of symptom onset.

Table 2 NINDS criteria	
Inclusion	Acute ischemic stroke
	Onset within 3 h
	NIHSS measurable deficit
	CT showing no hemorrhage
Exclusion	Previous stroke or head injury in previous 3 mo
	Major surgery in previous 14 d
	History of intracranial hemorrhage
	Systolic blood pressure >185 mm Hg
	Diastolic blood pressure >110 mmHg
	Rapidly improving or minor symptoms
	Symptoms suggestive of subarachnoid hemorrhage
	Gastrointestinal or urinary tract hemorrhage in previous 21 d
	Arterial puncture at noncompressible site in previous 7 d
	Presence of seizure at stroke onset
	Anticoagulant use
	Heparin use within 48 h AND elevated partial thromboplastin time
	Prothrombin times >15 sec
	Platelets <100,000/mm³
	Glucose <50 mg/dL or >400 mg/dL
	Aggressive treatment of blood pressure required

The Alteplase Thrombolysis for Acute Noninterventional Therapy in Ischemic Stroke (ATLANTIS) trial, Part A,[61] investigated the outcomes of tPA given within 6 hours of stroke onset. It was stopped early due to safety concerns. The results of Part A showed an increase in symptomatic intracerebral hemorrhage (11% in tPA, 0% in placebo, $P<.01$) and an increase in 90-day mortality (23% in tPA, 7% in placebo, $P<.01$), with no improvement in NIHSS at 30 days. Only 15% of the patients enrolled in Part A were treated before 3 hours, so the conclusion was made that these deleterious effects more accurately reflected initiation of therapy between 3 and 6 hours. Part B[62] was begun in its place, with tPA administration between 3 and 5 hours. Part B found that tPA administered between 3 and 5 hours after onset of symptoms provided no difference in excellent recovery (NIHSS 0–1) at 90 days and did not contribute to increased 90-day mortality (11% in tPA, 6.9% in placebo, $P = .09$).

With ECASS III, however, the timeline was definitively changed.[16] The initial study protocol looked at the effect of tPA when administered 3 to 4 hours after stroke onset. This timeline was extended midway through the study after publication of pooled analysis of prior tPA trials suggested a benefit through 4.5 hours.[63] When the primary endpoint was assessed using the modified Rankin criteria at three months, patients treated with tPA from 3 to 4.5 hours after onset were more likely to have favorable outcomes (Rankin 0–1) than those who received placebo. There was, in line with previous trials, an increased risk of intracerebral hemorrhage in the tPA arm (7.9% versus 3.5% for placebo, $P<.001$), but there was no difference in mortality between the two groups. A major difference in this trial, compared with the NINDS trial, was the addition of further exclusion criteria (**Table 3**). These additional exclusion criteria are: age greater than 80, NIHSS score greater than 25, patients taking oral anticoagulants (regardless of current INR), and those with a history of both prior stroke and diabetes mellitus. This excluded a large proportion of patients who would have been eligible for the NINDS trial, but who may be at a slightly higher risk for hemorrhage.

A meta-analysis of the 3- to 4.5-hour time window looked into the differences between the ATLANTIS and ECASS III trials.[64] A proposed theory for the lack of positive outcome with tPA in the ATLANTIS trial is the longer median time to treatment (4 hours 36 minutes versus 3 hours 59 minutes in ECASS III). This analysis confirmed the benefit of treatment up to 4.5 hours from symptom onset. Another updated pooled analysis of the eight major trials of tPA for acute stroke[65] found that not only is benefit seen when stroke is treated with tPA up to 4.5 hours after symptom onset, but also that earlier treatment within this window correlated with improved outcomes, providing evidence that every effort should be made to hasten time to thrombolytics. It also confirmed the previous finding that beyond 4.5 hours, the risk of bleeding outweighs the benefits of tPA.

Previously, intravenous tPA was estimated to cause hemorrhage in anywhere from 6% to 20% of patients.[59] In the pooled data analysis by Lees and colleagues,[65] the rate of large intracranial hemorrhage among the 8 trials was 5.2% in tPA patients and 1% of controls. In all tPA trials, care was taken to exclude patients with hemorrhage (via symptoms and/or imaging with CT/MRI), and repeat imaging was usually done between 22 and 36 hours, as well as at the physician's discretion.

The AHA/ASA updated the stroke guidelines in 2009[66] to recommend thrombolytic therapy for patients up to 4.5 hours from symptom onset (class 1, level of evidence B) with the caveat that the additional exclusion criteria for these patients be followed. Given the evidence that earlier treatment is beneficial, the goal door-to-needle time should remain 60 minutes. The approved dose of tPA is 0.9 mg/kg body weight with a maximum dose of 90 mg, given in two parts: 10% as a bolus over the first minute, and the remaining 90% over the next hour.

Table 3 ECASS III criteria	
Inclusion	Acute ischemic stroke Age 18–80 y Onset of stroke 3–4.5 h Stroke symptoms present for at least 30 min with no significant improvement before treatment
Exclusion	Intracranial hemorrhage Time of symptom onset unknown Symptoms rapidly improving or only minor before start of infusion Severe stroke as assessed clinically (eg, NIHSS score >25) or by appropriate imaging techniques[a] Seizure at onset of stroke Stroke or serious head trauma in previous 3 mo Combination of previous stroke and diabetes mellitus Administration of heparin within the 48 h preceding the onset of stroke, with an activated partial thromboplastin time at presentation exceeding the upper limit of the normal range Platelet <100,000/mm³ Systolic blood pressure >185 mm Hg Diastolic blood pressure >110 mm Hg Aggressive treatment of blood pressure required to reduce blood pressure to these limits Glucose <50 mg/dL or >400 mg/dL Symptoms suggestive of subarachnoid hemorrhage even if CT normal Oral anticoagulant use Major surgery or severe trauma in previous 3 mo Other major disorders associated with an increased risk of bleeding

[a] A severe stroke as assessed by imaging was defined as a stroke involving more than one third of the middle cerebral artery territory.

Endovascular

There are additional therapeutic options for the management of ischemic stroke. These include cerebral intra-arterial thrombolytics via percutaneous catheterization, combination intra-arterial and intravenous thrombolytics, and mechanical clot removal.

The Prolyse in Acute Cerebral Thromboembolism (PROACT) II trial,[67] which looked at intra-arterial prourokinase administration to patients with large MCA occlusions presenting within 6 hours, did show improved outcomes at 90 days (mRS of 0–2, $P = .04$) but also an increase in symptomatic intracranial hemorrhage within 24 hours.

Advantages of mechanical clot removal devices include a decreased risk of hemorrhage, a potentially longer treatment window, and ability to recanalize larger occluded vessels.[68] Just as endovascular treatment options are now preferred in the treatment of occlusive heart disease, it is logical to theorize similar positive results for ischemic cerebral disease. There have not been large randomized studies evaluating the safety and efficacy of these treatment modalities. Two clot retrieval devices, the Mechanical Embolus Removal in Cerebral Ischemia (MERCI; Concentric Medical, Incorporated, Mountain View, California) device and the Penumbra Suction Thrombectomy System (Penumbra, Incorporated, Alameda, California), have received FDA approval, and nonrandomized trials evaluating these devices have used therapeutic time windows of up to 8 hours.[69] There are limited data that suggest mechanical clot removal improves outcomes at 3 months.[70]

In a large meta-analysis it appears that recanalization may be an appropriate surrogate marker for improved outcomes,[71] whether by thrombolytics or mechanical devices. Vessel patency, by any means, was found to improve outcomes. The subset of patients who may be eligible for mechanical intervention include those presenting outside the intravenous tPA therapeutic window but within 8 hours of symptom onset, those with large vessel infarcts not appropriate for thrombolytics, and those who present to a facility with the appropriate consultants and resources available, including a neurointerventional radiologist, neurosurgeons, neurologists, and a stroke intensive care unit. Further discussion of endovascular techniques is available elsewhere in this issue.

SUMMARY

Progress continues to be made in the management of ischemic stroke. Emergency physicians are now able to offer stroke patients treatment options that improve functional outcomes. Since "time is brain," immediate recognition of ischemic stroke has become a top priority. Emergency physicians must be aware of the common presentations of stroke and be prepared to manage this disease quickly and efficiently.

Integrated systems expedite care of the stroke patient. Prehospital triage and notification allow activation of those systems before the patient arrives to the emergency department. Swift recognition of stroke syndromes, completion of the NIHSS score, care in ruling out stroke mimics, and expedited laboratory and radiology results are crucial to meeting guideline goals. Involvement of neurology and/or neurointerventional consultants should be simultaneous with evaluation of the patient.

Attention must be paid to optimum medical management of a stroke patient. For tPA candidates, blood pressure control should be initiated for pressures greater than 185/110 mm Hg. Blood glucose control should be considered for patients with admission values above 140 to 188 mg/dL.

All stroke patients should be considered candidates for lysis until they meet hard exclusion criteria. Thrombolytics should be considered before the evaluation is complete. A door-to-needle time of 60 minutes is the goal for treatment of ischemic stroke; however, a benefit can be seen in treatment given within 4.5 hours of symptom onset. Advanced imaging modalities may provide more detailed information that can expand a patient's treatment options. Endovascular therapies are evolving for patients who are not candidates for thrombolysis.

Ischemic stroke is a significant contributor to morbidity and mortality in the United States, and ameliorating disability is the goal of rapid stroke protocols. Ischemic stroke treatment is an active area of research, and there remains much to be discovered regarding the management of this important disease.

REFERENCES

1. Roger VL, Go AS, Lloyd-Jones DM, et al. Heart disease and stroke statistics—2011 update: a report from the American Heart Association. Circulation 2011;123(4):e18–209.
2. Tissue plasminogen activator for acute ischemic stroke. The National Institute of Neurological Disorders and Stroke rt-PA Stroke Study Group. N Engl J Med 1995;333(24):1581–7.
3. Fonarow GC, Saver JL, Saver JL, et al. Improving door-to-needle times in acute ischemic stroke: the design and rationale for the american heart association/american stroke association's target: stroke initiative. Stroke 2011;42(10):2983–9.

4. Ropper AH, Samuels MA, editors. Adams and victor's principles of neurology. 9th edition. The McGraw-Hill Companies, Inc; 2009.
5. Maulaz AB, Bezerra DC, Bogousslavsky J. Posterior cerebral artery infarction from middle cerebral artery infarction. Arch Neurol 2005;62(6):938–41.
6. Fisher CM. Capsular infarcts: the underlying vascular lesions. Arch Neurol 1979; 36(2):65–73.
7. Caplan LR. Intracranial branch atheromatous disease: a neglected, under-studied, and underused concept. Neurology 1989;39(9):1246–50.
8. Edlow JA, Newman-Toker DE, Savitz SI. Diagnosis and initial management of cerebellar infarction. Lancet Neurol 2008;7(10):951–64.
9. Nadeau S, Jordan J, Mishra S. Clinical presentation as a guide to early prognosis in vertebrobasilar stroke. Stroke 1992;23(2):165–70.
10. Sacco SE, Whisnant JP, Broderick JP, et al. Epidemiological characteristics of lacunar infarcts in a population. Stroke 1991;22(10):1236–41.
11. Fisher CM. Lacunar strokes and infarcts: a review. Neurology 1982;32(8):871–6.
12. Stam J. Thrombosis of the cerebral veins and sinuses. N Engl J Med 2005; 352(17):1791–8.
13. Ferro JM, Canhao P, Stam J, et al. Prognosis of cerebral vein and dural sinus thrombosis: results of the International Study on Cerebral Vein and Dural Sinus Thrombosis (ISCVT). Stroke 2004;35(3):664–70.
14. Saposnik G, Barinagarrementeria F, Brown RJ, et al. Diagnosis and management of cerebral venous thrombosis: a statement for healthcare professionals from the American Heart Association/American Stroke Association. Stroke 2011;42(4):1158–92.
15. Ferro JM, Canhao P, Stam J, et al. Delay in the diagnosis of cerebral vein and dural sinus thrombosis: influence on outcome. Stroke 2009;40(9):3133–8.
16. Hacke W, Kaste M, Bluhmki E, et al. Thrombolysis with alteplase 3 to 4.5 hours after acute ischemic stroke. N Engl J Med 2008;359(13):1317–29.
17. Jauch EC, Cucchiara B, Adeoye O, et al. Part 11: adult stroke: 2010 American Heart Association Guidelines for Cardiopulmonary Resuscitation and Emergency Cardiovascular Care. Circulation 2010;122(18 Suppl 3):S818–28.
18. Schwamm LH, Pancioli A, Acker JE 3rd, et al. Recommendations for the establishment of stroke systems of care: recommendations from the American Stroke Association's Task Force on the development of stroke systems. Stroke 2005; 36(3):690–703.
19. Kothari R, Barsan W, Brott T, et al. Frequency and accuracy of prehospital diagnosis of acute stroke. Stroke 1995;26(6):937–41.
20. Kothari RU, Pancioli A, Liu T, et al. Cincinnati Prehospital Stroke Scale: reproducibility and validity. Ann Emerg Med 1999;33(4):373–8.
21. Frendl DM, Strauss DG, Underhill BK, et al. Lack of impact of paramedic training and use of the Cincinnati Prehospital Stroke Scale on stroke patient identification and on-scene time. Stroke 2009;40(3):754–6.
22. Ramanujam P, Guluma KZ, Castillo EM, et al. Accuracy of stroke recognition by emergency medical dispatchers and paramedics—San Diego experience. Prehosp Emerg Care 2008;12(3):307–13.
23. Kidwell CS, Starkman S, Eckstein M, et al. Identifying stroke in the field: prospective validation of the Los Angeles Prehospital Stroke Screen (LAPSS). Stroke 2000;31(1):71–6.
24. Adams HP Jr, del Zoppo G, Alberts MJ, et al. Guidelines for the early management of adults with ischemic stroke: a guideline from the American Heart Association/American Stroke Association Stroke Council, Clinical Cardiology Council, Cardiovascular Radiology and Intervention Council, and the Atherosclerotic

Peripheral Vascular Disease and Quality of Care Outcomes in Research Interdisciplinary Working Groups: the American Academy of Neurology affirms the value of this guideline as an educational tool for neurologists. Stroke 2007;38(5): 1655–711.

25. Carter AM, Catto AJ, Mansfield MW, et al. Predictive variables for mortality after acute ischemic stroke. Stroke 2007;38(6):1873–80.

26. Singhal AB. Oxygen therapy in stroke: past, present, and future. Int J Stroke 2006;1(4):191–200.

27. Okumura K, Ohya Y, Maehara A, et al. Effects of blood pressure levels on case fatality after acute stroke. J Hypertens 2005;23(6):1217–23.

28. Vemmos KN, Tsivgoulis G, Spengos K, et al. U-shaped relationship between mortality and admission blood pressure in patients with acute stroke. J Intern Med 2004;255(2):257–65.

29. Leonardi-Bee J, Bath P, Phillips SJ, et al. Blood pressure and clinical outcomes in the international stroke trial. Stroke 2002;33(5):1315–20.

30. Castillo J, Leira R, Garcia MM, et al. Blood pressure decrease during the acute phase of ischemic stroke is associated with brain injury and poor stroke outcome. Stroke 2004;35(2):520–6.

31. Sandset EC, Bath PM, Boysen G, et al. The angiotensin-receptor blocker candesartan for treatment of acute stroke (SCAST): a randomised, placebo-controlled, double-blind trial. Lancet 2011;377(9767):741–50.

32. Mokin M, Kass-Hout T, Kass-Hout O, et al. Blood pressure management and evolution of thrombolysis-associated intracerebral hemorrhage in acute ischemic stroke. J Stroke Cerebrovasc Dis 2011 Jun 22. [Epub ahead of print].

33. Kallmunzer B, Kollmar R. Temperature management in stroke—an unsolved, but important topic. Cerebrovasc Dis 2011;31(6):532–43.

34. Groysman LI, Emanuel BA, Kim-Tenser MA, et al. Therapeutic hypothermia in acute ischemic stroke. Neurosurg Focus 2011;30(6):E17.

35. Ntaios G, Egli M, Faouzi M, et al. J-shaped association between serum glucose and functional outcome in acute ischemic stroke. Stroke 2010;41(10):2366–70.

36. Capes SE, Hunt D, Malmberg K, et al. Stress hyperglycemia and prognosis of stroke in nondiabetic and diabetic patients. Stroke 2001;32(10):2426–32.

37. Ahmed N, Davalos A, Eriksson N, et al. Association of admission blood glucose and outcome in patients treated with intravenous thrombolysis: results from the Safe Implementation of Treatments in Stroke International Stroke Thrombolysis Register (SITS-ISTR). Arch Neurol 2010;67(9):1123–30.

38. Bruno A, Levine SR, Frankel MR, et al. Admission glucose level and clinical outcomes in the NINDS rt-PA stroke trial. Neurology 2002;59(5):669–74.

39. Goldstein LB, Simel DL. Is this patient having a stroke? JAMA 2005;293(19): 2391–402.

40. Runchey S, McGee S. Does this patient have a hemorrhagic stroke? clinical findings distinguishing hemorrhagic stroke from ischemic stroke. JAMA 2010; 303(22):2280–6.

41. Goldstein LB, Samsa GP. Reliability of the National Institutes of Health Stroke Scale. Extension to non-neurologists in the context of a clinical trial. Stroke 1997;28(2):307–10.

42. Martin-Schild S, Albright KC, Tanksley J, et al. Zero on the NIHSS does not equal the absence of stroke. Ann Emerg Med 2011;57(1):42–5.

43. Woo D, Broderick JP, Kothari RU, et al. Does the National Institutes of Health Stroke Scale favor left hemisphere strokes? NINDS t-PA Stroke Study Group. Stroke 1999;30(11):2355–9.

44. Rost NS, Masrur S, Pervez MA, et al. Unsuspected coagulopathy rarely prevents IV thrombolysis in acute ischemic stroke. Neurology 2009;73(23):1957–62.
45. Cucchiara BL, Jackson B, Weiner M, et al. Usefulness of checking platelet count before thrombolysis in acute ischemic stroke. Stroke 2007;38(5):1639–40.
46. Walter S, Kostopoulos P, Haass A, et al. Point-of-care laboratory halves door-to-therapy-decision time in acute stroke. Ann Neurol 2011;69(3):581–6.
47. Latchaw RE. The roles of diffusion and perfusion MR imaging in acute stroke management. AJNR Am J Neuroradiol 1999;20(6):957–9.
48. Tomandl BF, Klotz E, Handschu R, et al. Comprehensive imaging of ischemic stroke with multisection CT. Radiographics 2003;23(3):565–92.
49. Kang DW, Chalela JA, Dunn W, et al. MRI screening before standard tissue plasminogen activator therapy is feasible and safe. Stroke 2005;36(9):1939–43.
50. Kidwell CS, Chalela JA, Saver JL, et al. Comparison of MRI and CT for detection of acute intracerebral hemorrhage. JAMA 2004;292(15):1823–30.
51. Fiebach JB, Schellinger PD, Jansen O, et al. CT and diffusion-weighted MR imaging in randomized order: diffusion-weighted imaging results in higher accuracy and lower interrater variability in the diagnosis of hyperacute ischemic stroke. Stroke 2002;33(9):2206–10.
52. Mullins ME, Schaefer PW, Sorensen AG, et al. CT and conventional and diffusion-weighted MR imaging in acute stroke: study in 691 patients at presentation to the emergency department. Radiology 2002;224(2):353–60.
53. Sorensen AG, Copen WA, Ostergaard L, et al. Hyperacute stroke: simultaneous measurement of relative cerebral blood volume, relative cerebral blood flow, and mean tissue transit time. Radiology 1999;210(2):519–27.
54. Keir SL, Wardlaw JM. Systematic review of diffusion and perfusion imaging in acute ischemic stroke. Stroke 2000;31(11):2723–31.
55. Murray V, Norrving B, Sandercock PA, et al. The molecular basis of thrombolysis and its clinical application in stroke. J Intern Med 2010;267(2):191–208.
56. Frendl A, Csiba L. Pharmacological and non-pharmacological recanalization strategies in acute ischemic stroke. Front Neurol 2011;2:32.
57. Hommel M, Boissel JP, Cornu C, et al. Termination of trial of streptokinase in severe acute ischaemic stroke. Lancet 1995;345(8941):57.
58. Donnan GA, Davis SM, Chambers BR, et al. Streptokinase for acute ischemic stroke with relationship to time of administration: Australian Streptokinase (ASK) Trial Study Group. JAMA 1996;276(12):961–6.
59. Hacke W, Kaste M, Fieschi C, et al. Intravenous thrombolysis with recombinant tissue plasminogen activator for acute hemispheric stroke. The European Cooperative Acute Stroke Study (ECASS). JAMA 1995;274(13):1017–25.
60. Hacke W, Kaste M, Fieschi C, et al. Randomised double-blind placebo-controlled trial of thrombolytic therapy with intravenous alteplase in acute ischaemic stroke (ECASS II). Second European-Australasian Acute Stroke Study Investigators. Lancet 1998;352(9136):1245–51.
61. Clark WM, Albers GW, Madden KP, et al. The rtPA (alteplase) 0- to 6-hour acute stroke trial, part A (A0276g): results of a double-blind, placebo-controlled, multicenter study. Thromblytic therapy in acute ischemic stroke study investigators. Stroke 2000;31(4):811–6.
62. Clark WM, Wissman S, Albers GW, et al. Recombinant tissue-type plasminogen activator (Alteplase) for ischemic stroke 3 to 5 hours after symptom onset. The ATLANTIS Study: a randomized controlled trial. Alteplase Thrombolysis for Acute Noninterventional Therapy in Ischemic Stroke. JAMA 1999;282(21):2019–26.

63. Hacke W, Donnan G, Fieschi C, et al. Association of outcome with early stroke treatment: pooled analysis of ATLANTIS, ECASS, and NINDS rt-PA stroke trials. Lancet 2004;363(9411):768–74.
64. Lansberg MG, Bluhmki E, Thijs VN. Efficacy and safety of tissue plasminogen activator 3 to 4.5 hours after acute ischemic stroke: a metaanalysis. Stroke 2009;40(7):2438–41.
65. Lees KR, Bluhmki E, von Kummer R, et al. Time to treatment with intravenous alteplase and outcome in stroke: an updated pooled analysis of ECASS, ATLANTIS, NINDS, and EPITHET trials. Lancet 2010;375(9727):1695–703.
66. del Zoppo GJ, Saver JL, Jauch EC, et al. Expansion of the time window for treatment of acute ischemic stroke with intravenous tissue plasminogen activator: a science advisory from the American Heart Association/American Stroke Association. Stroke 2009;40(8):2945–8.
67. Furlan A, Higashida R, Wechsler L, et al. Intra-arterial prourokinase for acute ischemic stroke. The PROACT II study: a randomized controlled trial. Prolyse in Acute Cerebral Thromboembolism. JAMA 1999;282(21):2003–11.
68. Meyers PM, Schumacher HC, Connolly ES Jr, et al. Current status of endovascular stroke treatment. Circulation 2011;123(22):2591–601.
69. Broderick JP. Endovascular therapy for acute ischemic stroke. Stroke 2009;40 (3 Suppl 1):S103–6.
70. Falluji N, Abou-Chebl A, Rodriguez Castro CE, et al. Reperfusion strategies for acute ischemic stroke. Angiology 2012;63(4):289–96 [Epub 2011 Jul 6].
71. Rha JH, Saver JL. The impact of recanalization on ischemic stroke outcome: a meta-analysis. Stroke 2007;38(3):967–73.

with variable sensitivity from 31% to 79%.[14,17] False-positive hyperdense MCA signs can occur in patients with higher hematocrits as well as patients with higher levels of calcification within blood vessel walls.[18]

Early ischemic changes that may be found on NCCT include loss of the gray-white interface in the basal ganglia and lentiform nucleus (obscuration of the lentiform nucleus) or the insular cortex (loss of the insular ribbon), hypodensity/hypoattenuation of the brain parenchyma, and focal and diffuse swelling of the cerebral parenchyma (**Fig. 2**).[16,19–23] Early ischemic changes are more likely to be seen in more severe stroke and in longer times from symptoms onset.[19] Obscuration of the lentiform nucleus and loss of the insular ribbon are the two most common early parenchymal findings on NCCT; these two regions of the brain are particularly vulnerable to early infarction because of tenuous blood supplies via end-arteries to the basal ganglia and a watershed arterial zone to the insular cortex.[9,21–23]

The significance of early ischemic changes on NCCT is highly debated.[6] Von Kummer and colleagues[16] initially showed that extensive parenchymal hypodensity or local brain swelling is highly predictive for fatal outcomes. In the European Cooperative Acute Stroke Study trials I and II, involvement of more than one-third of the MCA territory on NCCT was used as a criteria for exclusion from treatment with IV rt-PA because of the potential increased risk for hemorrhage and poor outcomes.[24,25] In contrast, Patel and colleagues[19] demonstrated that in the National Institute of Neurological Disorders and Stroke rt-PA stroke trial in 1995, signs of early ischemic changes on NCCT performed within 3 hours of time of symptom onset were not associated with an increased risk of adverse outcomes after treatment. Given this controversy, current prescribing information for IV rt-PA by the manufacturer Genetech does not list major early infarct signs on NCCT as a contradiction for treatment with IV rt-PA but does state that the risks associated with treatment may be increased in these patients and should be weighed against the anticipated benefits.[26]

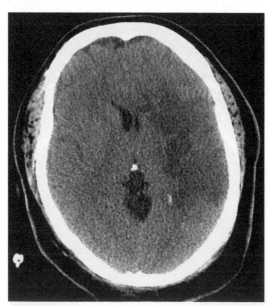

Fig. 2. Left MCA territory ischemic stroke on noncontrast brain CT depicting loss of the gray-white matter differentiation, hypoattenuation within the brain parenchyma, and focal swelling of the cerebral parenchyma with sulcal effacement.

CT Angiography

CTA is performed by administering an appropriately timed bolus of iodinated contrast through a peripheral large bore IV to maximize vascular opacification of the arterial circulation and acquire a volumetric dataset that can be processed to display 2-dimensional (2D) projectional or 3-dimensional (3D) volume-rendered images.[27,28] It is a minimally invasive tool for the imaging of vessels of the head and neck in patients presenting with suspected AIS, and advances in multidetector CT technology have made CTA the preferred noninvasive alternative to conventional catheter-based cerebral arteriography. Current CT scanners can provide a detailed evaluation of the extracranial and intracranial vasculature in less than 5 seconds by obtaining CTA from the aortic arch up to the circle of Willis with a single data acquisition and excellent isotropic spatial resolution.[9,29] CTA of the carotids can be performed from the aortic arch to the intracranial circulation to detect carotid artery disease with ulcerations or plaques that may account for an embolus or a stenosis limiting blood flow. CTA can evaluate the intracranial vessels for a site of occlusion or stenosis (**Fig. 3**)[29] and may guide diagnosis and therapy by aiding in the decision to administer an IV thrombolytic agent or have patients undergo intra-arterial thrombolysis with or without mechanical thrombolysis.[6]

With a single bolus of iodinated contrast material, CTA source images (CTA-SI) can provide a qualitative cerebral blood volume map that allows for the evaluation of tissue perfusion with resulting detection of the core of infarction and improved demonstration of tissue at risk for infarction compared with NCCT.[6] The benefit of CTA-SI is that, unlike other types of perfusion imaging, CTA-SI map the brain, do not rely on the interpretation of nonenhanced images, and are available immediately at the completion of the CTA because they do not require postprocessing. CTA-SI have been shown to be more sensitive that NCCT for the detection of early irreversible ischemia,[30] and lesion volumes seen on CTA-SI correlate with DWI abnormalities MRI.[31] CTA-SI seem to be as good as DWI at detecting acute ischemia with the exception of small strokes and strokes in the posterior fossa.[6]

CT Perfusion

CTP tracks a bolus of infused iodinated contrast material through brain tissue serially through time and, thus, allows a rapid, noninvasive, quantitative evaluation of dynamic brain perfusion. Because of a linear relationship between iodinated CT contrast

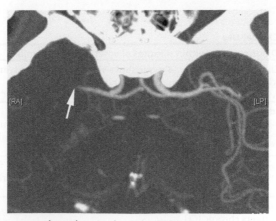

Fig. 3. CTA showing acute thrombus in the right MCA.

concentration and resulting imaging density, CTP is able to quantify cerebral blood volume, cerebral blood flow, and mean transit time required for blood to flow through brain tissue.[32] It allows for the investigation of alteration in cerebral perfusion in patients with suspected stroke and can delineate the ischemic core and ischemic penumbra. However, CTP requires repeatedly scanning the same portion of the brain over the time required for the contrast to pass through the tissue. As such, a large drawback to CTP is that scanners can only cover a limited number of slices of the brain, which does not allow for evaluating exact perfusion deficit volumes if they exceed the volume studied or for investigating areas of small perfusion deficit outside of the area chosen.[13] The 64-slice scanners allow for 8 or more perfusion brain slices thereby increasing the detection rate for AIS, and CTP has an overall sensitivity of about 75% for ischemic strokes with high specificity.[33] Newer, 256-slice and 360-slice CT scanners may offer whole-brain coverage.[34] However, CTP remains investigational because specific CTP and CTA criteria to identify patients who may benefit from thrombolysis has not been determined and the clinical value of the penumbral information that CTP provides has yet to be fully established.[34,35]

MAGNETIC RESONANCE IMAGING

Both CT and MRI are highly sensitive for the detection of intracranial hemorrhage, but MRI is much more sensitive than CT in detecting acute ischemic changes and, as such, is more accurate in diagnosing patients presenting with acute focal neurologic deficits.[11] Multimodal MRI can be used in the acute setting to evaluate and accurately diagnose patients with suspected acute stroke. It includes the following sequences: DWI, T2W/FLAIR, MRA, PWI, and GRE (**Table 2**).[5] Using these different imaging sequences, multimodal MRI is able to provide excellent anatomic detail of the brain; differentiate between ischemic and infarcted brain tissue; exclude ICH; and provide angiographic, spectroscopic, and perfusion information of the cerebral vasculature and tissue bed.[36] Additionally, MRI has a higher sensitivity and specificity than CT for the detection of other neurologic diseases that mimic acute stroke clinically, such as cerebral edema, vascular malformations, neoplasms, infection, inflammatory diseases, and toxic-metabolic disorders.[36] Multimodal MRI can be performed in 10 to 20 minutes, thus making it feasible within a 3-hour thrombolysis time window and competitive with multimodal CT regarding study acquisition time.[34,37]

Table 2
Multimodal MRI

Sequence	Clinical Use
DWI	Diagnoses AIS within minutes of onset of ischemic injury
FLAIR	Diagnoses subacute ischemic stroke within 3–8 h after symptom onset Identifies older ischemic strokes and small vessel disease May diagnose SAH (decreased accuracy compared with NCCT)
MRA	Identifies intracranial occlusions and stenosis Allows for the evaluation of the cranial circulation without IV contrast Evaluates for some secondary causes of ICH and vascular abnormalities in SAH (eg, aneurysms, arteriovenous malformations)
PWI	Depicts areas of brain tissue with reduced cerebral blood flow DWI-PWI mismatch may estimate an area of brain tissue at risk of infarction if blood flow is not restored
GRE	Diagnoses acute ICH Detects chronic ICH

In addition to the increased accuracy in diagnosing patients presenting with suspected acute stroke, MRI has the added advantage over CT of the lack of exposure to ionizing radiation. Disadvantages to MRI compared with CT include higher cost and lack of 24-hour availability of MRI at many hospitals.[36] Additionally, there are a few absolute contraindications to undergoing MRI, including the presence of cardiac pacemakers or certain ferromagnetic metallic implanted substances that may be displaced by the magnetic field. Additionally, approximately 5% of patients undergoing MRI experience claustrophobia,[38] which can increase difficulty in obtaining an MRI.

Diffusion Weighted Imaging and Apparent Diffusion Coefficient

DWI is able to depict areas of acute brain ischemia using the random motion of water molecules within living tissues (Brownian motion). In the first few minutes of vascular occlusion during an ischemic stroke, cerebral ischemia leads to the disruption in energy metabolism causing a failure of the sodium-potassium adenosine triphosphatase pump and other ion pumps. This membrane channel failure leads to a loss of ionic gradients and a net shift of water molecules into the intracellular compartment with resultant swelling of the cells (ie, cytotoxic edema). This edema leads to a reduction of the extracellular space thereby reducing the Brownian molecular motion of water molecules in this space. The reduction of Brownian molecular motion in infarcted tissue caused by reduced water diffusion can be rapidly detected as a hyperintense lesion on DWI (**Fig. 4**)[39,40] within minutes of vessel occlusion and the onset of ischemia.[41] This decrease in water diffusion in ischemic brain tissue can be measured quantitatively with the apparent diffusion coefficient (ADC).[39] Additionally, because DWI is T2 based, shine through of high T2W abnormalities, such as chronic stroke or vasogenic edema, may be misinterpreted as acute ischemia on DWI. The correlation of DWI with the ADC map, which demonstrates restricted diffusion of water molecules as low intensity, greatly increases the specificity of DWI in AIS.[6,40] Hyperacute ischemic brain lesions have increased signal intensity on DWI and decreased signal intensity on ADC (**Fig. 5**).[41]

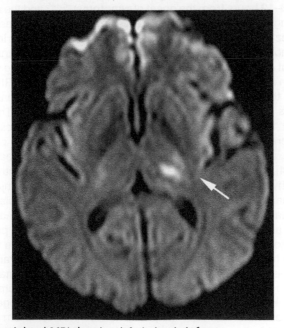

Fig. 4. Diffusion-weighted MRI showing left thalamic infarct.

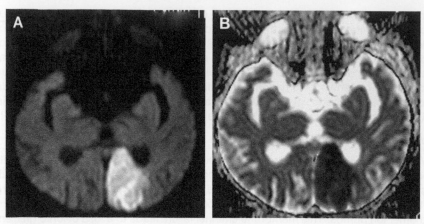

Fig. 5. Hyperacute left occipital ischemic stroke with increased signal intensity on DWI (*A*) and decreased signal intensity on corresponding ADC (*B*).

DWI is the imaging modality of choice for the timely and accurate diagnosis of AIS. It has been shown to detect physiologic changes within 15 minutes of ischemic injury in both experimental animal models and in patients presenting with AIS.[41] Moseley and colleagues[42] first demonstrated that acute occlusion of the MCA in animal models produced DWI hyperintensity in ischemic regions within 45 minutes after the onset of ischemia and much sooner than conventional T2W images. In the mid-1990s, research on DWI in AIS progressed to human patients when DWI showed improved stroke diagnostics with infarcts appearing sooner on DWI than on conventional MRI.[43,44]

Multiple studies have confirmed the increased sensitivity and accuracy of DWI over CT and conventional MRI in identifying areas of ischemia in patients presenting with early AIS (within 6–12 hours from the onset of symptoms),[45–49] and the overall accuracy of DWI diagnosing acute ischemia improves as time of symptom onset decreases. A study by González and colleagues[47] showed that in patients in whom imaging was performed within 6 hours of symptom onset, DWI was 100% sensitive and 100% specific in the diagnosis of AIS. In a subset of patients who underwent imaging within 3 hours of symptom onset in a prospective study by Chalela and colleagues, MRI was found to be superior to CT in the blinded imaging diagnosis of AIS, with 73% sensitivity and 92% specificity versus 12% sensitivity and 100% specificity for CT. The overall false-negative rate for DWI in this study was 17%, and factors associated with false-negative DWI were brainstem location of stroke, time of symptom onset to imaging less than 3 hours, and mild stroke with a low National Institutes of Health Stroke Scale score (less than 4). None of the false-negative DWI cases were positive on CT.[11]

Although DWI hyperintensity appears within minutes of ischemic injury, DWI lesions may be at least partially reversible in the early phase of brain ischemia, and the size of the DWI abnormality does not necessarily reflect irreversibly damaged tissue.[39] A study by Fiehler and colleagues[50] evaluating 68 patients with AIS presenting within 6 hours of symptom onset who underwent serial MRI examinations found that 20% of these patients had ADC normalization in greater than 5 mL of brain tissue on MRI performed between days 5 to 8. All patients with partial ADC normalization demonstrated at least partial tissue reperfusion, and tissue with a more severe initial decrease in ADC was less likely to demonstrate normalization. This study suggests brain tissue with initially decreased ADC, especially within 3 hours of symptom onset, may still represent salvageable tissue at risk that could benefit from thombolytics.[50] As such,

DWI is no longer thought to be a simple indicator of tissue irreversible infarction but a more complex variable that requires additional careful study. Additionally, other cerebral pathologic conditions can cause false-positive DWI through restricted diffusion, such as infection, inflammatory conditions, and certain tumors.[6]

T2-Weighted and Fluid-Attenuated Inversion Recovery

On T2W and FLAIR images, ischemic infarction appears as a hyperintense lesion usually within the first 3 to 8 hours after stroke onset.[9] FLAIR imaging provides an advantage over the more conventional T2W imaging in that it nulls the signal from the cerebrospinal fluid (CSF) while providing a heavily T2W image of the brain parenchyma. The suppression of the CSF signal allows for better detection of acute infarcts, especially the cortical gray matter infarcts.[51–53] Although superior to T2W imaging, the sensitivity of FLAIR is lower than DWI for the diagnosis of AIS and increases with increased time from symptom onset. A recent study of patients with AIS presenting within 6 hours of symptom onset by Thomalla and colleagues[53] found that patients with a mismatch with a positive DWI and negative FLAIR were likely to have been imaged within 3 hours of symptom onset with a 93% specificity and 94% positive predictive value. As such, a DWI positive–FLAIR negative mismatch may be useful in identifying patients with an unknown time of stroke onset who may benefit from thrombolysis,[53] which is described in more detail later in this article.

Unique signs of AIS may be identified on FLAIR imaging within the first 24 hours after the onset of symptoms. Acute infarcts may appear on FLAIR imaging as swollen cortical gyri with increased signal intensity. These hyperintense, swollen gyri represent cytotoxic edema and correspond to areas of ischemia seen on DWI.[52,54] Increased signal intensity in the lumen of vessels may be observed on FLAIR imaging in patients with AIS.[52,54,55] This finding is known as the hyperintense vessel sign (HVS) or arterial hyperintensity and has been found to be associated with large vessel occlusion or severe stenosis.[55] The exact pathophysiology of the HVS remains unclear; it may represent slow moving or stationary blood, intraluminal thrombus, or retrograde collateral circulation. The sensitivity of HVS is highest during the first 6 hours of onset, and the presence of HVS accompanied by ischemic changes on DWI indicates impending infarction and should prompt consideration of revascularization and flow augmentation strategies. Occasionally, the HVS on FLAIR imaging may be the earliest ischemic change noted on MRI and may precede diffusion abnormalities.[54–57] In patients presenting with stroke symptoms who are not suffering an ischemic event, FLAIR imaging may also depict hyperintense intracranial hemorrhagic lesions as well as cerebral venous thrombosis.[54] Additionally, both T2W and FLAIR imaging can be used to assess for older ischemic strokes and the extent of small vessel disease.[39]

MR Angiography

Noncontrast 3D time-of-flight (TOF) MRA is the mainstay of intracranial arterial evaluation by MRI allowing for high-spatial-resolution isotropic imaging of the cranial vascular system. TOF MRA is based on the differences between protons in stationary tissue, which are saturated by repeated radiofrequency excitations and produce low signal intensity, and the high signal from fresh unsaturated protons that move into the imaging slab via the cranial arteries between each excitation pulse. It produces flow-dependent luminal imaging, and visualization of the vessel wall is limited.[58] TOF MRA can be both 2D and 3D and has the benefits of not requiring a carefully timed contrast agent to produce, being easily repeatable,[59] and not exposing patients to radiation. However, compared with CTA, TOF MRA has limitations because of its sensitivity to patient motion artifact and flow artifact, which may result in the

more accurate than CT in the detection of chronic hemorrhage. These results were confirmed in a prospective study by Chalela and colleagues[11] comparing NCCT with MRI in the evaluations of consecutive ED patients presenting with suspected acute stroke. 217 of the 356 patients in this study had a final diagnosis of acute stroke with MRI being similar to CT for the detection of acute ICH and better than CT for the detection of acute ischemia and chronic hemorrhage.[11]

GRE is superior to CT for the detection of chronic hemorrhage, particularly cerebral microbleeds (CMBs), which are small collections of hemosiderin deposits that are foci of past hemorrhages. CMBs appear as small, round, black dots on GRE. Recent evidence suggests that CMBs may be a marker of underlying vascular pathologic conditions, particularly hypertensive vasculopathy and cerebral amyloid angiopathy. The presence as well as the number of CMBs may predict future risk of symptomatic ICH in patients who have suffered a primary ICH or AIS.[71] However, a recent large multicenter study of 570 patients with AIS who were treated with IV rt-PA found no significant absolute increase in the risk of symptomatic ICH in patients with CMBs identified on initial GRE versus those without.[72] Presently, whether CMBs should affect clinical decision making remains an area of future research.[71]

Much like the hyperdense artery signs seen on CT (described earlier in this article), a hypointense signal in a cerebral artery on GRE may indicate acute thrombosis in the vessel. The presence of this susceptibility sign on GRE indicating thrombotic occlusion may help to guide treatment. However, it is important to be sure to distinguish between the hypointense signal indicating vessel occlusion and a hypointense region of intraparenchymal hemorrhage.[73,74]

MRI in Patients with Unknown Time of Symptom Onset

AIS occurs unwitnessed or during sleep in as many as 25% of all patients.[75] However, treatment with IV rt-PA is time dependent, with late treatment being ineffective or harmful[76]; clinical guidelines exclude treatment with IV thrombolysis in patients in whom time of onset is unknown and last seen normal is outside of 3 to 4.5 hours.[5] Many stroke investigators and clinicians advocate the use of imaging criteria to make treatment decisions in patients presenting with AIS whose exact time of onset of symptoms is unknown or is outside of the approved 3- to 4.5-hour treatment window for thrombolytic therapy. These stroke experts argue that treatment should be based on a tissue clock over a ticking clock to select patients who would most likely respond favorably to extended time window therapy.[41]

Multiparametric MRI has been suggested as a means to identify patients with AIS who are likely to be within a 3- to 4.5-hour time window and benefit from IV thrombolysis. Because DWI lesions can be detected with minutes from onset of ischemia and FLAIR is sensitive for subacute ischemia but cannot usually detect hyperacute ischemic lesions within the first few hours, one MRI combination sequence that may be favorable for detecting AIS within 3 to 4.5 hours from ischemia onset is a DWI-positive with FLAIR-negative mismatch. A recent large multicenter observational study, Predictive Value of FLAIR and DWI for the identification of patients with Acute Ischemic Stroke within 4.5 hours of symptom onset, showed that DWI-FLAIR mismatch can be used to identify patients within 4.5 hours of symptom onset with 78% specificity and 83% positive predictive value. The investigators concluded that patients with an acute ischemic lesion detected on DWI but not on FLAIR imaging are likely to be within a time window in which thrombolysis is safe and effective.[77]

In addition to MRI sequences potentially serving as a surrogate for duration of ischemia, it is hypothesized that imaging may be used as a marker of tissue salvageability. As described previously, it has been proposed that the use of DWI-PWI mismatch identifies tissue that may be saved and can be used in triaging patients that may benefit from thrombolytic therapy, even if their symptom onset is outside of 3 to 4.5 hours. Multiple trials have used DWI and PWI mismatch for inclusion criteria with variable results and the clinical utility remains yet unknown and investigational.

Currently, several interventional trials in patients with stroke with unknown symptom onset are proposed with varying trial designs and imaging enrollment criteria. It is hoped that the results of these trials in conjunction with future research will provide imaging techniques that allow additional insight into tissue injury and salvageability so as to safely and effectively extend treatment with IV thrombolysis to patients with an unclear onset of symptoms who may benefit from therapy.[78]

INTRACEREBRAL HEMORRHAGE

ICH is defined as spontaneous, nontraumatic bleeding into the brain parenchyma (**Fig. 7**).[79] Patients suffering from ICH present similarly to patients with AIS with sudden onset focal neurologic deficits. Certain clinical findings are more likely to be associated with ICH over AIS, including loss of consciousness, coma, neck stiffness, seizure accompanying the neurologic deficit, diastolic blood pressure greater than 110 mm Hg, vomiting, and headache. Although these additional characteristics are more often associated with patients with ICH, many patients with ICH lack any of these distinctive findings. The diagnosis of ICH, and its differentiation from AIS, cannot be made clinically and requires definitive neuroimaging.[80] Guidelines on the management of ICH from both the AHA Stroke Council and the European Stroke Initiative state that rapid neuroimaging is required to distinguish ICH from AIS.[81,82]

As discussed previously, both CT and MRI can be used in the initial evaluation of patients presenting with possible ICH. NCCT is thought to be 100% sensitive for detecting clinically relevant acute hemorrhage and is considered the criterion standard for diagnosing ICH.[81] As discussed previously, GRE is as sensitive as NCCT for the detection of acute intracranial hemorrhage, and MRI is a more accurate imaging

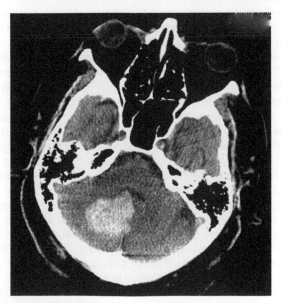

Fig. 7. Acute ICH in the right cerebellum on noncontrast brain CT.

modality for patients presenting with possible acute stroke given its increased sensitivity for AIS and chronic hemorrhage.[10,11] However, certain patient and hospital factors, such as the availability of MRI, patient contraindications, and patient medical instability, may make obtaining an MRI impossible or impractical in the acute setting.[83]

Once ICH is diagnosed, additional neuroimaging may be performed to identify patients at risk for hematoma expansion and evaluate for secondary causes of ICH that may be amenable to treatment or intervention. CTA and contrast-enhanced CT may identify patients at risk for hematoma expansion. Contrast extravasation into the hematoma on a CTA or contrast-enhanced CT appears as a small, enhancing focus within the hematoma that is known as a spot sign. Patients found to have a spot sign are at a high risk for hematoma expansion[84,85] and the clinical use of this radiological marker is an area of active research. MRI, MRA, MR venogram, and CTA may be useful to exclude secondary causes of ICH, such as aneurysms, tumors, cerebral venous thrombosis, arteriovenous malformations, or fistulas.[81] Nonlobar hemorrhages involving the putamen, globus pallidus, thalamus, internal capsule, periventricular white matter, pons, and cerebellum in patients with known hypertension are often, although not exclusively, caused by hypertensive vasculopathy. Patients with hemorrhages in other locations, including isolated intraventricular hemorrhage, and younger patients or patients without a history of hypertension are at a higher risk for secondary ICH.[82,86]

SUBARACHNOID HEMORRHAGE

Headache is a common complaint accounting for approximately 2% of all ED visits.[87] Although most headaches are caused by primary headache disorders, such as migraines or tension-type headaches, some acute headaches are caused by serious pathologic conditions with significant morbidity and mortality, such as SAH. In fact, of all patients presenting to the ED with headache, approximately 1% had SAH.[88] Many patients with SAH present with sudden-onset severe headache with variably associated signs or symptoms, including nausea and vomiting, stiff neck, loss of consciousness, or focal neurologic deficits. Given the variability in types of headaches and inconsistency in associated symptoms, misdiagnosis or delayed diagnosis in SAH is common, with the most common diagnostic error being the failure to obtain proper imaging.[89]

The first best diagnostic study to obtain in the workup of SAH is the NCCT (**Fig. 8**).[88–90] NCCT should be obtained with very thin cuts through the base of the brain so as not to miss small collections of blood.[88] NCCT is highly accurate in the diagnosis of SAH, but the probability of detecting SAH on NCCT is proportional to the amount of hemorrhage and the time from hemorrhage onset.[89] The accuracy of the NCCT declines over time because of the circulation of the CSF and the resulting dilution and breakdown of the blood.[90] In the first 12 hours after hemorrhage, the sensitivity of NCCT for SAH is 98% to 100%, declining to 93% at 24 hours and to 57% to 85% 6 days after the onset of SAH.[89] As technology improves, modern multidetector CT scanners show improving sensitivity for the diagnosis of SAH. A recent study by Perry and colleagues[91] evaluating the sensitivity of modern third-generation CT for diagnosis of SAH showed an overall sensitivity of NCCT of 93% and 100% sensitivity for patients who underwent NCCT within 6 hours of headache onset. However, until further large studies confirm the 100% sensitivity of modern and early NCCT, patients being evaluated for SAH with negative NCCT should undergo lumbar puncture to look for small amounts of xanthochromia or blood in the CSF.[92]

MRI is constantly advancing and shows promise for the evaluation and diagnosis of SAH.[90] Both proton-density–weighted images and FLAIR images have shown to

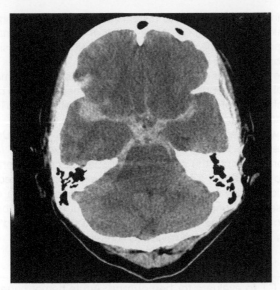

Fig. 8. Acute SAH as seen on noncontrast brain CT.

reliably detect hyperacute SAH in patients with NCCT-positive SAH.[93,94] However, in patients with NCCT-negative SAH that was diagnosed by lumbar puncture, FLAIR MRI was found to be infrequently positive.[95] Additionally, on FLAIR, CSF pulsation artifacts can mimic blood in the third and fourth ventricles and around the cisterns and give a false-positive result.[34] No large prospective studies of MR diagnosis in patients with suspected SAH exist, and CT remains the study of choice because of its speed, availability, and ease of diagnosis.[6,90]

Once SAH is diagnosed, the intracranial vessels should be imaged as soon as possible after patient stabilization to evaluate for aneurysms or other vascular abnormalities that may be intervened on. In nontraumatic SAH, 80% of cases are caused by ruptured intracranial aneurysms, 10% by nonaneurysmal venous peri-mesencephalic hemorrhages, and the remaining 10% by other vascular lesions, tumors, and other less common causes.[90] Imaging of the intracranial vessels for aneurysms can be accomplished by DSA, CTA, or MRA, with CTA and DSA having a higher accuracy rate than MRA.[6] It has been shown that 3D TOF MRA and CE-MRA have a sensitivity and specificity similar to those of CTA for the detection of intracerebral aneurysms that are 5 mm or larger and have a lower sensitivity for the detection of aneurysms smaller than 5 mm.[59]

READING A NONCONTRAST HEAD CT SCAN

As described previously, the "2010 American Heart Association Guidelines for Cardiopulmonary Resuscitation and Emergency Cardiovascular Care" for patients with acute stroke recommend that an NCCT should be completed within 25 minutes of the patients' arrival and interpreted within 45 minutes of ED arrival.[12] Given the time-sensitive nature of acute stroke, emergency physicians should have the ability to interpret an NCCT and identify acute pathologic conditions in patients presenting with acute onset of focal neurologic deficits. The following section briefly reviews a rapid and thorough manner with which to read an NCCT to evaluate for significant pathologic conditions that requires emergent intervention. As with any radiologic interpretation, a knowledge of the basic normal anatomy and function of the brain parenchyma, its vasculature, and its ventricles and cisterns is necessary in interpreting potential pathologic conditions on a head CT. A full review of cranial neuroanatomy is beyond the scope of this article, and the clinician is encouraged to review basic neuroanatomy as is necessary for his or her understanding.

In reviewing the NCCT, the emergency physician must be systematic in his or her approach. Several different approaches to reading the head CT have been recommended, including a checklist of items to follow when interpreting a NCCT[96] or a central to peripheral approach on each image from the first through the last.[97] To aid the emergency physician who does not frequently review head CT scans, Dr Perron and his colleagues[98,99] developed the mnemonic "*blood can be very bad*" in which the first letter of each word prompts the clinician to evaluate a certain portion of the head CT for pathologic conditions. This method has been demonstrated to work in the ED, and the clinician may use the mnemonic when examining a cranial CT scan because the presence of one finding does not rule out additional pathologic conditions. The components of the mnemonic "blood can be very bad", devoloped by Dr Perron and his colleagues[99] are reviewed subsequently.

Blood

Review the head CT to evaluate for hemorrhage. Acute hemorrhage appears hyperdense (bright white) on a CT (**Fig. 9**A). Hemorrhage appears isodense around 1 to 2 weeks and hypodense by 2 to 3 weeks. Evaluate the head CT for epidural hematomas

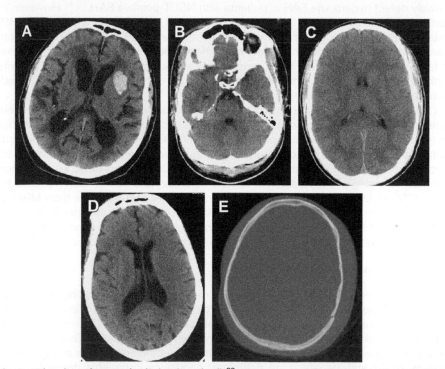

Fig. 9. "Blood can be very bad" (as described).[99] Acute intracerebral blood in the left front lobe appears as a hyperintense (*bright white*) lesion (*A*). Cisterns are CSF collections jacketing the brain; suprasellar and circummesencephalic cisterns on NCCT (*B*). Appearance of normal brain on NCCT (*C*). Lateral ventricles on NCCT (*D*). Left parietal skull fracture on bone windows of NCCT (*E*).

(lens shaped), subdural hematomas (crescent shaped), intraparenchymal hemorrhage, intraventricular hemorrhage, SAH, and extracranial hemorrhage.

Cisterns

Cisterns are CSF collections jacketing the brain (see **Fig. 9**B). Four key cisterns, circummesencephalic, suprasellar, quadrigeminal, and sylvian, must be examined for blood, asymmetry, and effacement (evidence of increased intracranial pressure).

Brain

Normal brain parenchyma is inhomogeneous where cortical gray matter is denser than subcortical white matter (see **Fig. 9**C). When examining the brain parenchyma, the clinician should look for symmetry, gray-white differentiation, evidence of shift, and evidence of hyperdensity or hypodensity. Hyperdensity is caused by blood, calcification, or IV contrast. Hypodensity may be caused by pneumocephalus, ischemia, edema, or tumor.

Ventricles

Pathologic processes can cause hydrocephalus or compression/shift of the ventricular system (see **Fig. 9**D). Hydrocephalus is usually first evident in the dilation of the temporal horns.

Bone

Fractures may occur at any portion of the skull, and the presence of a skull fracture should increase suspicion for an intracranial injury (see **Fig. 9**E). The diagnosis of a linear skull fracture can be confusing because of sutures, and the clinician should compare with the other side of the skull to look for suture symmetry versus fracture.

REFERENCES

1. Roger VL, Go AS, Lloyd-Jones DM, et al. Heart disease and stroke statistics–2012 update: a report from the American Heart Association. Circulation 2012; 125(1):e2–220.
2. Tissue plasminogen activator for acute ischemic stroke. The National Institute of Neurological Disorders and Stroke rt-PA Stroke Study Group. N Engl J Med 1995; 333(24):1581–7.
3. Hacke W, Kaste M, Bluhmki E, et al. Thrombolysis with alteplase 3 to 4.5 hours after acute ischemic stroke. N Engl J Med 2008;359(13):1317–29.
4. Del Zoppo GJ, Saver JL, Jauch EC, et al. Expansion of the time window for treatment of acute ischemic stroke with intravenous tissue plasminogen activator: a science advisory from the American Heart Association/American Stroke Association. Stroke 2009;40(8):2945–8.
5. Adams HP Jr, del Zoppo G, Alberts MJ, et al. Guidelines for the early management of adults with ischemic stroke: a guideline from the American Heart Association/American Stroke Association Stroke Council, Clinical Cardiology Council, Cardiovascular Radiology and Intervention Council, and the Atherosclerotic Peripheral Vascular Disease and Quality of Care Outcomes in Research Interdisciplinary Working Groups: the American Academy of Neurology affirms the value of this guideline as an educational tool for neurologists. Stroke 2007;38(5):1655–711.
6. Latchaw RE, Alberts MJ, Lev MH, et al. Recommendations for imaging of acute ischemic stroke: a scientific statement from the American Heart Association. Stroke 2009;40(11):3646–78.

7. Ginde AA, Foianini A, Renner DM, et al. Availability and quality of computed tomography and magnetic resonance imaging equipment in U.S. emergency departments. Acad Emerg Med 2008;15(8):780–3.

8. Scharf J, Brockmann MA, Daffertshofer M, et al. Improvement of sensitivity and interrater reliability to detect acute stroke by dynamic perfusion computed tomography and computed tomography angiography. J Comput Assist Tomogr 2006;30(1):105–10.

9. Leiva-Salinas C, Wintermark M. Imaging of acute ischemic stroke. Neuroimaging Clin N Am 2010;20(4):455–68.

10. Kidwell CS, Chalela JA, Saver JL, et al. Comparison of MRI and CT for detection of acute intracerebral hemorrhage. JAMA 2004;292(15):1823–30.

11. Chalela JA, Kidwell CS, Nentwich LM, et al. Magnetic resonance imaging and computed tomography in emergency assessment of patients with suspected acute stroke: a prospective comparison. Lancet 2007;369(9558):293–8.

12. Jauch EC, Cucchiara B, Adeoye O, et al. Part 11: adult stroke: 2010 American Heart Association guidelines for cardiopulmonary resuscitation and emergency cardiovascular care. Circulation 2010;122(18 Suppl 3):S818–28.

13. Lovblad KO, Baird AE. Computed tomography in acute ischemic stroke. Neuroradiology 2010;52(3):175–87.

14. Leys D, Pruvo JP, Godefroy O, et al. Prevalence and significance of hyperdense middle cerebral artery in acute stroke. Stroke 1992;23(3):317–24.

15. Schuknecht B, Ratzka M, Hofmann E. The "dense artery sign"–major cerebral artery thromboembolism demonstrated by computed tomography. Neuroradiology 1990;32(2):98–103.

16. von Kummer R, Meyding-Lamade U, Forsting M, et al. Sensitivity and prognostic value of early CT in occlusion of the middle cerebral artery trunk. AJNR Am J Neuroradiol 1994;15(1):9–15 [discussion 16–18].

17. Tomsick TA, Brott TG, Chambers AA, et al. Hyperdense middle cerebral artery sign on CT: efficacy in detecting middle cerebral artery thrombosis. AJNR Am J Neuroradiol 1990;11(3):473–7.

18. Rauch RA, Bazan C 3rd, Larsson EM, et al. Hyperdense middle cerebral arteries identified on CT as a false sign of vascular occlusion. AJNR Am J Neuroradiol 1993;14(3):669–73.

19. Patel SC, Levine SR, Tilley BC, et al. Lack of clinical significance of early ischemic changes on computed tomography in acute stroke. JAMA 2001; 286(22):2830–8.

20. von Kummer R, Holle R, Gizyska U, et al. Interobserver agreement in assessing early CT signs of middle cerebral artery infarction. AJNR Am J Neuroradiol 1996; 17(9):1743–8.

21. Truwit CL, Barkovich AJ, Gean-Marton A, et al. Loss of the insular ribbon: another early CT sign of acute middle cerebral artery infarction. Radiology 1990;176(3): 801–6.

22. Sarikaya B, Provenzale J. Frequency of various brain parenchymal findings of early cerebral ischemia on unenhanced CT scans. Emerg Radiol 2010;17(5):381–90.

23. Tomura N, Uemura K, Inugami A, et al. Early CT finding in cerebral infarction: obscuration of the lentiform nucleus. Radiology 1988;168(2):463–7.

24. Hacke W, Kaste M, Fieschi C, et al. Intravenous thrombolysis with recombinant tissue plasminogen activator for acute hemispheric stroke. The European Cooperative Acute Stroke Study (ECASS). JAMA 1995;274(13):1017–25.

25. Hacke W, Kaste M, Fieschi C, et al. Randomised double-blind placebo-controlled trial of thrombolytic therapy with intravenous alteplase in acute ischaemic stroke

(ECASS II). Second European-Australasian Acute Stroke Study Investigators. Lancet 1998;352(9136):1245–51.

26. Inc. GU. Activase Prescribing Information. Accessed April 28, 2012.

27. Chen MY, Pope TL, Ott DJ. Basic radiology. 2nd edition. New York: McGraw Hill Medical; 2011. Available at: http://www.accessmedicine.com/resourceTOC.aspx?resourceID=75. Accessed April 28, 2012.

28. Adam A, Dixon AK, Grainger RG, et al. consulting editors. In: Adam A, Dixon AK, Grainger RG, et al, editors. Grainger and Allison's diagnostic radiology: A textbook of medical imaging. 5th edition. Edinburgh (United Kingdom): Churchill Livingstone; 2008.

29. Prokop M. Multislice CT angiography. Eur J Radiol 2000;36(2):86–96.

30. Camargo EC, Furie KL, Singhal AB, et al. Acute brain infarct: detection and delineation with CT angiographic source images versus nonenhanced CT scans. Radiology 2007;244(2):541–8.

31. Schramm P, Schellinger PD, Fiebach JB, et al. Comparison of CT and CT angiography source images with diffusion-weighted imaging in patients with acute stroke within 6 hours after onset. Stroke 2002;33(10):2426–32.

32. Eastwood JD, Lev MH, Provenzale JM. Perfusion CT with iodinated contrast material. AJR Am J Roentgenol 2003;180(1):3–12.

33. Brainin M, Heiss WD, Heiss S. Textbook of stroke medicine. Cambridge (United Kingdom): Cambridge University Press; 2010.

34. Merino JG, Warach S. Imaging of acute stroke. Nat Rev Neurol 2010;6(10): 560–71.

35. Kohrmann M, Schellinger PD. Acute stroke triage to intravenous thrombolysis and other therapies with advanced CT or MR imaging: pro MR imaging. Radiology 2009;251(3):627–33.

36. Xavier AR, Qureshi AI, Kirmani JF, et al. Neuroimaging of stroke: a review. South Med J 2003;96(4):367–79.

37. Schellinger PD, Jansen O, Fiebach JB, et al. Feasibility and practicality of MR imaging of stroke in the management of hyperacute cerebral ischemia. AJNR Am J Neuroradiol 2000;21(7):1184–9.

38. Edelman RR, Warach S. Magnetic resonance imaging (1). N Engl J Med 1993; 328(10):708–16.

39. Kloska SP, Wintermark M, Engelhorn T, et al. Acute stroke magnetic resonance imaging: current status and future perspective. Neuroradiology 2010;52(3):189–201.

40. Schaefer PW, Grant PE, Gonzalez RG. Diffusion-weighted MR imaging of the brain. Radiology 2000;217(2):331–45.

41. Wu O, Nentwich L, Chutinet A, et al. Diffusion in acute stroke. In: Jones DK, editor. Diffusion MRI: theory, methods, and applications. New York, Oxford (United Kingdom): Oxford University Press; 2011. p. 518–28.

42. Moseley ME, Cohen Y, Mintorovitch J, et al. Early detection of regional cerebral ischemia in cats: comparison of diffusion- and T2-weighted MRI and spectroscopy. Magn Reson Med 1990;14(2):330–46.

43. Warach S, Chien D, Li W, et al. Fast magnetic resonance diffusion-weighted imaging of acute human stroke. Neurology 1992;42(9):1717–23.

44. Warach S, Gaa J, Siewert B, et al. Acute human stroke studied by whole brain echo planar diffusion-weighted magnetic resonance imaging. Ann Neurol 1995; 37(2):231–41.

45. Barber PA, Darby DG, Desmond PM, et al. Identification of major ischemic change. Diffusion-weighted imaging versus computed tomography. Stroke 1999;30(10): 2059–65.

46. Lovblad KO, Laubach HJ, Baird AE, et al. Clinical experience with diffusion-weighted MR in patients with acute stroke. AJNR Am J Neuroradiol 1998;19(6): 1061–6.
47. Gonzalez RG, Schaefer PW, Buonanno FS, et al. Diffusion-weighted MR imaging: diagnostic accuracy in patients imaged within 6 hours of stroke symptom onset. Radiology 1999;210(1):155–62.
48. Mullins ME, Schaefer PW, Sorensen AG, et al. CT and conventional and diffusion-weighted MR imaging in acute stroke: study in 691 patients at presentation to the emergency department. Radiology 2002;224(2):353–60.
49. Fiebach JB, Schellinger PD, Jansen O, et al. CT and diffusion-weighted MR imaging in randomized order: diffusion-weighted imaging results in higher accuracy and lower interrater variability in the diagnosis of hyperacute ischemic stroke. Stroke 2002;33(9):2206–10.
50. Fiehler J, Knudsen K, Kucinski T, et al. Predictors of apparent diffusion coefficient normalization in stroke patients. Stroke 2004;35(2):514–9.
51. Brant-Zawadzki M, Atkinson D, Detrick M, et al. Fluid-attenuated inversion recovery (FLAIR) for assessment of cerebral infarction. Initial clinical experience in 50 patients. Stroke 1996;27(7):1187–91.
52. Noguchi K, Ogawa T, Inugami A, et al. MRI of acute cerebral infarction: a comparison of FLAIR and T2-weighted fast spin-echo imaging. Neuroradiology 1997; 39(6):406–10.
53. Thomalla G, Rossbach P, Rosenkranz M, et al. Negative fluid-attenuated inversion recovery imaging identifies acute ischemic stroke at 3 hours or less. Ann Neurol 2009;65(6):724–32.
54. Makkat S, Vandevenne JE, Verswijvel G, et al. Signs of acute stroke seen on fluid-attenuated inversion recovery MR imaging. AJR Am J Roentgenol 2002;179(1): 237–43.
55. Kamran S, Bates V, Bakshi R, et al. Significance of hyperintense vessels on FLAIR MRI in acute stroke. Neurology 2000;55(2):265–9.
56. Maeda M, Yamamoto T, Daimon S, et al. Arterial hyperintensity on fast fluid-attenuated inversion recovery images: a subtle finding for hyperacute stroke undetected by diffusion-weighted MR imaging. AJNR Am J Neuroradiol 2001; 22(4):632–6.
57. Toyoda K, Ida M, Fukuda K. Fluid-attenuated inversion recovery intraarterial signal: an early sign of hyperacute cerebral ischemia. AJNR Am J Neuroradiol 2001;22(6):1021–9.
58. Miyazaki M, Lee VS. Nonenhanced MR angiography. Radiology 2008;248(1): 20–43.
59. Bowen BC. MR angiography versus CT angiography in the evaluation of neuro-vascular disease. Radiology 2007;245(2):357–60 [discussion: 360–1].
60. Yoo AJ, Pulli B, Gonzalez RG. Imaging-based treatment selection for intravenous and intra-arterial stroke therapies: a comprehensive review. Expert Rev Cardiovasc Ther 2011;9(7):857–76.
61. Bash S, Villablanca JP, Jahan R, et al. Intracranial vascular stenosis and occlusive disease: evaluation with CT angiography, MR angiography, and digital subtraction angiography. AJNR Am J Neuroradiol 2005;26(5):1012–21.
62. Tomanek AI, Coutts SB, Demchuk AM, et al. MR angiography compared to conventional selective angiography in acute stroke. Can J Neurol Sci 2006; 33(1):58–62.
63. Rosen BR, Belliveau JW, Vevea JM, et al. Perfusion imaging with NMR contrast agents. Magn Reson Med 1990;14(2):249–65.

64. Hacke W, Albers G, Al-Rawi Y, et al. The Desmoteplase in Acute Ischemic Stroke Trial (DIAS): a phase II MRI-based 9-hour window acute stroke thrombolysis trial with intravenous desmoteplase. Stroke 2005;36(1):66–73.

65. Furlan AJ, Eyding D, Albers GW, et al. Dose Escalation of Desmoteplase for Acute Ischemic Stroke (DEDAS): evidence of safety and efficacy 3 to 9 hours after stroke onset. Stroke 2006;37(5):1227–31.

66. Hacke W, Furlan AJ, Al-Rawi Y, et al. Intravenous desmoteplase in patients with acute ischaemic stroke selected by MRI perfusion-diffusion weighted imaging or perfusion CT (DIAS-2): a prospective, randomised, double-blind, placebo-controlled study. Lancet Neurol 2009;8(2):141–50.

67. Albers GW, Thijs VN, Wechsler L, et al. Magnetic resonance imaging profiles predict clinical response to early reperfusion: the diffusion and perfusion imaging evaluation for understanding stroke evolution (DEFUSE) study. Ann Neurol 2006; 60(5):508–17.

68. Davis SM, Donnan GA, Parsons MW, et al. Effects of alteplase beyond 3 h after stroke in the Echoplanar Imaging Thrombolytic Evaluation Trial (EPITHET): a placebo-controlled randomised trial. Lancet Neurol 2008;7(4):299–309.

69. Linfante I, Llinas RH, Caplan LR, et al. MRI features of intracerebral hemorrhage within 2 hours from symptom onset. Stroke 1999;30(11):2263–7.

70. Fiebach JB, Schellinger PD, Gass A, et al. Stroke magnetic resonance imaging is accurate in hyperacute intracerebral hemorrhage: a multicenter study on the validity of stroke imaging. Stroke 2004;35(2):502–6.

71. Greenberg SM, Vernooij MW, Cordonnier C, et al. Cerebral microbleeds: a guide to detection and interpretation. Lancet Neurol 2009;8(2):165–74.

72. Fiehler J, Albers GW, Boulanger JM, et al. Bleeding risk analysis in stroke imaging before thromboLysis (BRASIL): pooled analysis of T2*-weighted magnetic resonance imaging data from 570 patients. Stroke 2007;38(10):2738–44.

73. Chalela JA, Haymore JB, Ezzeddine MA, et al. The hypointense MCA sign. Neurology 2002;58(10):1470.

74. Rovira A, Orellana P, Alvarez-Sabin J, et al. Hyperacute ischemic stroke: middle cerebral artery susceptibility sign at echo-planar gradient-echo MR imaging. Radiology 2004;232(2):466–73.

75. Hill MD, Frayne R. Stroke on awakening and the tissue window for thrombolysis. Lancet Neurol 2011;10(11):951–2.

76. Lees KR, Bluhmki E, von Kummer R, et al. Time to treatment with intravenous alteplase and outcome in stroke: an updated pooled analysis of ECASS, ATLANTIS, NINDS, and EPITHET trials. Lancet 2010;375(9727):1695–703.

77. Thomalla G, Cheng B, Ebinger M, et al. DWI-FLAIR mismatch for the identification of patients with acute ischaemic stroke within 4.5 h of symptom onset (PRE-FLAIR): a multicentre observational study. Lancet Neurol 2011;10(11):978–86.

78. Wu O, Schwamm LH, Sorensen AG. Imaging stroke patients with unclear onset times. Neuroimaging Clin N Am 2011;21(2):327–44, xi.

79. Qureshi AI, Tuhrim S, Broderick JP, et al. Spontaneous intracerebral hemorrhage. N Engl J Med 2001;344(19):1450–60.

80. Runchey S, McGee S. Does this patient have a hemorrhagic stroke?: clinical findings distinguishing hemorrhagic stroke from ischemic stroke. JAMA 2010; 303(22):2280–6.

81. Morgenstern LB, Hemphill JC 3rd, Anderson C, et al. Guidelines for the management of spontaneous intracerebral hemorrhage: a guideline for healthcare professionals from the American Heart Association/American Stroke Association. Stroke 2010;41(9):2108–29.

82. Steiner T, Kaste M, Forsting M, et al. Recommendations for the management of intracranial haemorrhage - part I: spontaneous intracerebral haemorrhage. The European Stroke Initiative Writing Committee and the Writing Committee for the EUSI Executive Committee. Cerebrovasc Dis 2006;22(4):294–316.

83. Singer OC, Sitzer M, du Mesnil de Rochemont R, et al. Practical limitations of acute stroke MRI due to patient-related problems. Neurology 2004;62(10): 1848–9.

84. Goldstein JN, Fazen LE, Snider R, et al. Contrast extravasation on CT angiography predicts hematoma expansion in intracerebral hemorrhage. Neurology 2007;68(12):889–94.

85. Wada R, Aviv RI, Fox AJ, et al. CT angiography "spot sign" predicts hematoma expansion in acute intracerebral hemorrhage. Stroke 2007;38(4):1257–62.

86. Zhu XL, Chan MS, Poon WS. Spontaneous intracranial hemorrhage: which patients need diagnostic cerebral angiography? A prospective study of 206 cases and review of the literature. Stroke 1997;28(7):1406–9.

87. Goldstein JN, Camargo CA Jr, Pelletier AJ, et al. Headache in United States emergency departments: demographics, work-up and frequency of pathological diagnoses. Cephalalgia 2006;26(6):684–90.

88. Edlow JA, Caplan LR. Avoiding pitfalls in the diagnosis of subarachnoid hemorrhage. N Engl J Med 2000;342(1):29–36.

89. Bederson JB, Connolly ES Jr, Batjer HH, et al. Guidelines for the management of aneurysmal subarachnoid hemorrhage: a statement for healthcare professionals from a special writing group of the Stroke Council, American Heart Association. Stroke 2009;40(3):994–1025.

90. Edlow JA, Malek AM, Ogilvy CS. Aneurysmal subarachnoid hemorrhage: update for emergency physicians. J Emerg Med 2008;34(3):237–51.

91. Perry JJ, Stiell IG, Sivilotti ML, et al. Sensitivity of computed tomography performed within six hours of onset of headache for diagnosis of subarachnoid haemorrhage: prospective cohort study. BMJ 2011;343:d4277.

92. Edlow JA, Panagos PD, Godwin SA, et al. Clinical policy: critical issues in the evaluation and management of adult patients presenting to the emergency department with acute headache. Ann Emerg Med 2008;52(4):407–36.

93. Wiesmann M, Mayer TE, Yousry I, et al. Detection of hyperacute subarachnoid hemorrhage of the brain by using magnetic resonance imaging. J Neurosurg 2002;96(4):684–9.

94. Fiebach JB, Schellinger PD, Geletneky K, et al. MRI in acute subarachnoid haemorrhage; findings with a standardised stroke protocol. Neuroradiology 2004; 46(1):44–8.

95. Mohamed M, Heasly DC, Yagmurlu B, et al. Fluid-attenuated inversion recovery MR imaging and subarachnoid hemorrhage: not a panacea. AJNR Am J Neuroradiol 2004;25(4):545–50.

96. Mettler FA, ScienceDirect (Online service). Essentials of radiology. 2nd edition. Philadelphia: Elsevier Saunders; 2005. Available at: http://www.mdconsult.com/public/book/view?title=Mettler:+Essentials+of+Radiology. Accessed April 28, 2012.

97. Yousem DM, Grossman RI. Neuroradiology: the requisites. 3rd edition. Philadelphia: Mosby/Elsevier; 2010.

98. Perron AD, Huff JS, Ullrich CG, et al. A multicenter study to improve emergency medicine residents' recognition of intracranial emergencies on computed tomography. Ann Emerg Med 1998;32(5):554–62.

99. Perron AD. How to read a head CT scan. In: Adams JM, editor. Emergency medicine. Philadelphia, London: Saunders; 2008. p. 753–63.

Vertigo, Vertebrobasilar Disease, and Posterior Circulation Ischemic Stroke

Jeffrey I. Schneider, MD*, Jonathan S. Olshaker, MD

KEYWORDS

- Vertigo • Vertebrobasilar disease • Posterior circulation ischemic stroke • Dizziness

KEY POINTS

- Patients with dizziness frequently present to the emergency department. The cause of the complaint ranges from the benign to the life threatening.
- Ischemia of structures supplied by the posterior circulation may present in a more subtle fashion than those affecting the anterior circulation.
- Posterior circulation ischemia rarely presents as a single symptom.
- The classic presentation of those with posterior circulation ischemia has been described as crossed findings with cranial nerve findings on the side of the lesion and long tract (eg, motor or sensory) findings on the contralateral side.
- Data regarding the cause and treatment of posterior circulation stroke has lagged behind that of anterior circulation stroke.

An estimated 7.5 million patients with dizziness are seen each year in ambulatory care settings.[1] It is one of the most common principal complaints in the emergency department (ED), responsible for 2.5% of all ED visits.[2] Benign paroxysmal positional vertigo, thought to be caused by loose particles in the semicircular canals, is the most common cause of vertigo, with an incidence estimated to be 107 cases per 100 000 population per year.[3] Dizziness in older individuals is associated with a variety of cardiovascular, neurosensory, and psychiatric conditions and with the use of multiple medications.[4] Among patients older than 60 years, 20% have experienced dizziness severe enough to affect their daily activity.[5] In a study of 1000 outpatients, dizziness was the third most common complaint. Vertigo is defined more clearly as a sensation of disorientation in space combined with a sensation of motion. Dizziness and imbalance are most commonly seen with peripheral processes but they can be the only clinical manifestations of a central life threat.

Department of Emergency Medicine, Boston Medical Center, Dowling 1 South, 1 Boston Medical Center Place, Boston, MA 02118, USA
* Corresponding author.
E-mail address: jeffrey.schneider@bmc.org

Emerg Med Clin N Am 30 (2012) 681–693
http://dx.doi.org/10.1016/j.emc.2012.06.004
0733-8627/12/$ – see front matter © 2012 Elsevier Inc. All rights reserved.

This article focuses on diagnosis and treatment when stroke and other central neurologic processes are in the differential.

PATHOPHYSIOLOGY

A complaint of dizziness is an imprecise term. The ED physician may think that these patients will be difficult to interview and that the condition will be problematic to diagnose and treat. But in reality, most of these patients have an organic basis for symptoms that can be successfully identified and treated. The diagnostic process is consistently based on 2 basic concepts: deciding whether patients have true vertigo and, if vertigo exists, deciding whether the cause is a central or peripheral neurologic entity.[6]

The maintenance of equilibrium and awareness of the body in relationship to its surroundings depend on the interaction of 3 systems: visual, proprioceptive, and vestibular. The eyes, muscles, joints, and otic labyrinths continuously supply information about the position of the body. Visual impulses, mediated through the higher brain centers, provide information about body position in space. Impulses from proprioceptors of the joints and muscles supply data about the relative positions of the parts of the body. Impulses from the neck are of special importance in relating the position of the head to the rest of the body. The sense organs of the visual, vestibular, and proprioceptive systems are connected with the cerebellum by way of the vestibular nuclei in the brainstem. Any disease that interrupts the integration of these 3 systems may give rise to symptoms of vertigo and disequilibrium.

DIAGNOSTIC APPROACH
Differential Considerations

Patients use the term *dizzy* to describe a variety of experiences, including sensations of motion, weakness, fainting, light-headedness, unsteadiness, and depression. To clarify the picture, it is often helpful to have patients describe the sensation without using the word *dizzy*. True vertigo may be defined as a sensation of disorientation in space combined with a sensation of motion. There is a hallucination of movement either of the self (subjective vertigo) or the external environment (objective vertigo). Descriptions of light-headedness or feeling faint are more consistent with presyncope. The differential diagnosis for these patients should include hypovolemia, dysrhythmias, myocardial infarction, sepsis, drug side effects, and pulmonary embolism. For some patients, dizziness is simply a metaphor for malaise, representing a variety of other causes, such as anemia, viral illness, or depression.

If patients have true vertigo, the clinician must determine whether the cause is a peripheral lesion (eg, of the inner ear) or a central process, such as cerebrovascular disease or a neoplasm. In most cases, peripheral disorders are benign and central processes are more serious. Occasionally, as in the case of a cerebellar hemorrhage, immediate therapeutic intervention is indicated. Acute suppurative labyrinthitis is the only cause of peripheral vertigo that requires urgent intervention.

Pivotal Findings

History
The medical history is the most important source of information. A first key question is, does true vertigo exist? Do patients have a sensation of disorientation in space or a sensation of motion? The sensation of spinning usually indicates a vestibular disorder. Some nausea, vomiting, pallor, and perspiration accompany almost all but the mildest forms of vertigo. The presence of these symptoms without vertigo should suggest a different cause. The labyrinth has no effect on the level of consciousness.

Patients should not have an associated change in mentation or syncope. A sensation of imbalance often accompanies vertigo, but true instability, disequilibrium, or ataxia makes a central process more likely.[7] The symptom of imbalance in most cases should warrant a workup for stroke.

Because nystagmus accompanies acute vertigo, it is often helpful to ask members of the patients' family if they have noted any unusual eye movements during the dizzy spells. This question is especially important in children unable to offer a concise history.[8] Occasionally, patients may be able to describe a flickering or oscillating visual field immediately after a change in position, such as rolling over in bed. In addition, interviewing family and other witnesses can often uncover evidence suggesting seizures, syncope, or imbalance unrelated to feelings of vertigo.

The *time of onset* and the *duration of vertigo* are important clues to the cause. Episodic vertigo that is severe, lasts several hours, and has symptom-free intervals between episodes suggests a peripheral labyrinth disorder. Vertigo produced primarily by a change in position also suggests a peripheral disorder. Vestibular neuronitis and benign positional vertigo fit this pattern.

The presence of *auditory symptoms* suggests a peripheral cause of the vertigo, as in middle and inner ear problems, or a peripheral cause that progresses centrally, such as an acoustic neuroma. The abnormally hearing ear is usually the side of end-organ disturbance. Progressive unilateral hearing loss of several months duration may be the earliest symptom of an acoustic neuroma. Tinnitus occurs in most patients with acoustic neuroma and, along with vertigo, is what often prompts patients to seek medical attention. Another peripheral process, Meniere disease, can present with the characteristic triad of hearing loss, vertigo, and tinnitus.

Are there associated neurologic symptoms? Patients or family members should be questioned about the time of onset of ataxia or gait disturbances. Ataxia of recent and sudden onset suggests cerebellar hemorrhage or infarction in the distribution of the posterior inferior cerebellar artery or the superior cerebellar artery. The salient feature of chronic cerebellar disorders is a slowly progressive ataxia. True ataxia may be difficult to discern from the unsteadiness that occurs when patients with significant vertigo attempt to walk.

Vertiginous symptoms are common after head injuries. The presence of recent head or neck trauma should be explored because vertiginous symptoms are common after both.[9,10] Head injuries can cause vertigo occasionally from intracerebral injury and more commonly from labyrinth concussion. Neck injuries can cause vertigo from strain of muscle proprioceptors. In addition, a vertebral artery injury has been seen resulting from activities, such as chiropractic manipulation and even hair shampooing with marked hyperextension in a salon.[11]

It has clearly been shown that isolated vertigo can be the only initial symptom of cerebellar and other posterior circulation bleeds, transient ischemic attacks (TIAs), and infarction.[12–14] One study showed that emergency physicians often did not make the correct diagnosis in patients with validated strokes or TIAs that presented with only vertigo.[7] Identifying these individuals is without a doubt the most important and difficult challenge for clinicians taking care of patients with vertigo. Most patients with isolated dizziness do not have TIA or stroke but the risk of not identifying the few that do is significant for ultimate patient outcomes. Stroke has been seen in 3.2% of patients with a dizziness syndrome but only 0.7% of those with isolated dizziness had a stroke.[7] A recent study also showed less than 1 in 500 patients discharged with a diagnosis of dizziness or vertigo experienced a major vascular event in the month after discharge.[15] In addition, a cross-sectional study of the National Hospital Ambulatory Medical Care Survey suggests significant overuse of computed tomography (CT) in low-risk patients.[16] Risk-factor assessment and symptom patterns can be extremely helpful in deciding which patients warrant imaging, neurologic consultation, and admission. Older age, male sex, and the presence of hypertension, coronary artery disease, diabetes mellitus, and atrial fibrillation puts patients at a higher risk for having an acute stroke as the cause of their symptoms. In addition, frequent episodes lasting only minutes or prolonged episodes of a day or more are more often associated with central processes.[7,12,13] One retrospective study showed that emergency physicians often failed to chart the triggers and the duration of dizziness, information that could potentially lead to increased likelihood of a more serious cause of symptoms.[17] Also, as previously mentioned, the symptom of imbalance raises the likelihood of TIA and stroke.

Past medical history

Many medications have direct vestibulotoxicity. The most commonly encountered are the aminoglycosides, anticonvulsants, alcohols, quinine, quinidine, and minocycline. In addition, caffeine and nicotine can have wide-ranging autonomic effects that may exacerbate vestibular symptoms. The history of past and present illnesses should be explored, with specific questioning about the existence of diabetes, drug or alcohol use, and the risk factors mentioned earlier.

Physical Examination

Vital signs

In some cases, pulses and blood pressure should be checked in both arms. Most patients with subclavian steal syndrome, which can also cause vertebrobasilar artery insufficiency, have pulse or systolic blood pressure differences between the two arms.

Head and neck

Carotid or vertebral artery bruits suggest atherosclerosis. The neck is auscultated along the course of the carotid artery from the supraclavicular area to the base of the skull.

Vertigo can be caused by impacted cerumen or a foreign object in the ear canal. Accumulation of fluid behind the eardrum as a result of a middle ear infection may cause mild vertigo, as can occlusion of the eustachian tubes associated with an upper respiratory tract infection. A perforated or scarred eardrum may indicate a perilymphatic fistula, especially if the history includes previous trauma.

The examination of the eyes is key in assessing patients with vertigo or disequilibrium. The focus is on any pupillary abnormalities indicating third cranial nerve or descending sympathetic tract involvement or optic disk signs of early increased intracranial pressure. Extraocular movements should be assessed carefully. Relatively subtle ocular movement abnormalities can be the only clue to a cerebellar hemorrhage. A sixth cranial nerve palsy ipsilateral to the hemorrhage may result from early brainstem compression by the expanding hematoma. Internuclear ophthalmoplegia is recognized when the eyes are in a normal position on straight-ahead gaze but on eye movement the adducting eye (cranial nerve III) is weak or shows no movement while the abducting eye (cranial nerve VI) moves normally, although often displaying a coarse nystagmus. This finding indicates an interruption of the medial longitudinal fasciculus on the side of the third cranial nerve weakness.

Abnormal nystagmus is the cardinal sign of inner ear disease and the principal objective evidence of abnormal vestibular function. In nystagmus, patients have difficulty maintaining the conjugate deviation of the eyes or have a postural control imbalance of eye movements.

The abnormal jerk nystagmus of inner ear disease consists of slow and quick components. The eyes slowly drift in the direction of the diseased hypoactive ear, then quickly jerk back to the intended direction of gaze. Positional nystagmus, induced by rapidly changing the position of the head, strongly suggests an organic vestibular disorder. A central nervous system cause of positional nystagmus should be considered when the pattern of nystagmus is persistent down beating, pure torsional, or when it is refractory to repositioning maneuvers. The characteristics of nystagmus are one of the most valuable tools for distinguishing peripheral from central causes of vertigo.

Positional testing
If nystagmus is not present at rest, positional testing can be helpful in determining its existence and characteristics. In the Hallpike maneuver, patients are moved quickly from an upright seated position to a supine position and the head is turned to one side and extended (to a head-down posture) approximately 30° from the horizontal plane off the end of the stretcher. The eyes should be observed for nystagmus, and patients should be queried for the occurrence of symptoms. This test should be repeated with the head turned to the other side. Positive elicitation of symptoms and signs to one side or the other generally indicates a vestibular pathologic condition on that same side. This test should be performed with caution if vertebrobasilar insufficiency is suggested because sudden twisting movements theoretically might dislodge atheromatous plaques.

Neurologic examination
The presence of cranial nerve deficits suggests a space-occupying lesion in the brainstem or cerebellopontine angle. The corneal reflex is a sensory cranial nerve (V) and motor cranial nerve (VII) circuit. Its diminution or absence can be one of the early signs of an acoustic neuroma. Vertigo caused by eighth cranial nerve involvement is likely to be accompanied by a unilateral hearing loss. Patients cannot hear a tuning fork when it is held alongside the affected ear but they can hear it when it is held against the mastoid process. The involvement of the eighth cranial nerve suggests an acoustic tumor. Seventh cranial nerve involvement causes facial palsy that affects the side of the face. In supranuclear facial paralysis, the forehead is spared because these muscles receive bilateral cortical innervation.

Patients should be evaluated specifically for evidence of cerebellar dysfunction. This examination must be performed in bed and standing because truncal ataxia may be occult on testing of the limbs in bed and may become obvious only when patients have to sit, stand, or walk unaided. Dysmetria is the inability to arrest a muscular movement at the desired point. Dysmetria should be assessed using finger-to-finger/finger-to-nose pointing and heel-to-shin testing, and dysdiadochokinesia (an inability to perform coordinated muscular movement smoothly) is assessed with rapid alternating movements. The gait must be evaluated when patients give a history suggesting ataxia, although examination may be impossible during an attack of vertigo. Any marked abnormality (eg, consistent falling or a grossly abnormal gait) should suggest a central lesion, especially in patients whose vertiginous symptoms have subsided. The main features of a cerebellar gait are a wide base (separation of legs), unsteadiness, irregularity of steps, tremor of the trunk, and lurching from side to side. The unsteadiness is most prominent on arising quickly from a sitting position, turning quickly, or stopping suddenly while walking. Patients with gait ataxia cannot perform heel-to-toe walking.

Ancillary Testing

Most routine laboratory testing is not helpful in the evaluation of patients with vertigo. A finger-stick blood glucose test should be performed in most cases because hypoglycemia can present as vertigo.[18] Blood counts and blood chemistries are sometimes helpful when it is difficult to distinguish whether dizziness is vertigo or near syncope. An electrocardiogram should be obtained if there is any possibility of myocardial ischemia or dysrhythmia.

Radiologic imaging

If cerebellar hemorrhage, cerebellar infarction, or other central lesions are suggested, emergent CT or magnetic resonance imaging (MRI) of the brain is indicated. MRI, when available, has become the diagnostic modality of choice when cerebellar processes other than acute hemorrhage are possible. MRI is particularly useful for the diagnosis of acoustic neuromas and for sclerotic and demyelinating lesions of the white matter, as seen in multiple sclerosis. Acute vertigo by itself does not warrant urgent CT or MRI in all patients, particularly patients in whom a clear picture of peripheral vertigo emerges. But as mentioned earlier, many studies strongly support the use of imaging in patients of advanced age or at risk for cerebrovascular disease.[7,12,13,19] CT, although often useful for identifying hemorrhage, is insensitive for acute stroke presentations, especially for infarction within the posterior fossa. MRI with MR angiography (MRA) is considered a much more sensitive modality and should be performed quickly in patients with changing neurologic signs and symptoms, suggesting impending posterior circulation occlusion. The use of these modalities is discussed in more depth in the subsequent sections.

Audiology and electronystagmography are helpful in the follow-up evaluation of patients with vertigo. Audiology can locate the anatomic site of a lesion causing vertigo. Electronystagmography is a collection of examinations that, when abnormal, suggest vestibular dysfunction but do not yield the specific diagnosis.

Posterior circulation stroke The clinical presentations of patients with posterior circulation ischemia can be vague and may overlap significantly with many frequently seen ED complaints. As described previously, approximately 7.5 million individuals with dizziness are seen in ambulatory care settings in the United States annually.[1] Importantly, less than 25% of cases are thought to result from a central cause.[20] As with many other ED scenarios, the emergency physician is faced with the challenge of identifying the few patients with concerning pathologic conditions from the many with less serious causes of illness.

Epidemiology

Posterior circulation strokes (PCS) account for approximately 20% to 30%[21-23] of all strokes, and the clinical manifestations of the disease can be varied. Although some patients may experience mild, intermittent brainstem symptoms (thought to arise from fluctuations in posterior circulation blood flow), others may unfortunately become locked-in, which is a result of basilar artery or bilateral vertebral artery occlusion in which patients retain full awareness and cognition but only have movements of their eyelids or eyes. Similarly, the mortality of PCS ranges from as low as 3.6% (at 30 days)[24] to more than 90% for those who are locked-in.[25]

Anatomy

Classically, the posterior circulation consists of the vertebral arteries, the basilar artery, the posterior cerebral arteries, and their branches. The vertebral arteries arise from the subclavian arteries and course through the vertebral foramina of the sixth through second cervical vertebrae before traversing the foramen magnum. At the level of the pontomedullary junction, the vertebrals join to create the basilar artery. Distally, the basilar artery divides into the posterior cerebral arteries and, finally, the posterior communicating artery in the circle of Willis. Although there is significant variability in the exact arterial anatomy of the posterior circulation, these arteries supply the brainstem, the thalamus, the hippocampus, the cerebellum, and portions of the occipital and temporal lobes.[26]

ED Presentation

Ischemia of structures supplied by the posterior circulation may present in a more subtle fashion than those affecting the anterior circulation. For example, in contrast to disease affecting the middle cerebral artery, obvious speech, motor, and sensory deficits are often not the dominant presenting feature. In one large series of patients with confirmed PCS, dizziness, dysarthria, headache, nausea/vomiting, and blurred vision were the most common presenting symptoms, whereas unilateral limb weakness, gait ataxia, unilateral limb ataxia, dysarthria, and nystagmus were the most common presenting signs.[27] In another series of patients with posterior circulation events, vertigo, unsteadiness, dysarthria, and nausea/vomiting were the most common presenting symptoms, whereas the most common neurologic signs included facial palsy, ataxia, focal weakness, and nystagmus.[28] Posterior circulation ischemia rarely presents as a single symptom. Rather, depending on the location of the ischemia, patients present with a constellation of symptoms and signs; less than 1% of patients in one series had a single presenting symptom or sign.[24] Patients may also present with significant alterations in their level of consciousness ranging from mild lethargy to frank coma if areas, such as the reticular activating system, are involved.[27,29]

The classic presentation of those with posterior circulation ischemia has been described as crossed findings with cranial nerve findings on the side of the lesion and long tract (eg, motor or sensory) findings on the contralateral side. Signs that may indicate vertebrobasilar ischemia include internuclear ophthalmoplegia, unreactive pupils, skew deviation, hemianopia, and cortical blindness.[27]

The exact constellation of symptoms and findings depends on the precise location of the infarct; commonly described syndromes include Wallenberg syndrome (nystagmus, vertigo, ataxia, hoarseness, dysphagia); Anton syndrome (somnolence, memory defects, confusion, visual hallucinations with bilateral loss of vision with unawareness or denial of blindness, vertical gaze paralysis, skew deviation of the eyes); Weber syndrome (ipsilateral oculomotor palsy with contralateral hemiplegia); and Dejerine-Roussy syndrome (contralateral hemisensory loss of all modalities).

Importantly, patients presenting with symptoms consistent with a TIA of the posterior circulation are thought to be at a high risk for early recurrent ischemic events. Although the risk of subsequent early stroke on patients with carotid artery stenosis has been well documented, only in recent years has a similar phenomenon been reported in those with stenosis of the vertebrobasilar system. The development of contrast-enhanced MRA and contrast CT angiography (CTA) has enabled investigators to noninvasively study the posterior circulation, and the risk of recurrent PCS (after initial stroke or TIA) is thought to be as high as 30.5%.[22,30]

ED Diagnosis

As with many other conditions, the ED physician must maintain a high level of suspicion to identify patients with evidence of posterior circulation ischemia. Patient complaints may be vague, and neurologic abnormalities may be subtle; the astute clinician must rely heavily on a thorough history and physical examination with particular focus on the cranial nerves, eye movements, and cerebellar findings.

Endovascular therapy

The successful use of percutaneous transluminal angioplasty in coronary and renal arteries led to attempts to use similar techniques for diseases of the posterior cerebral circulation. Unfortunately, however, complications, such as plaque disruption resulting in distal emboli and arterial vasospasm, have limited the utility of this practice. One retrospective study of 21 patients who had failed medical therapy, had poor collateral flow, were deemed high risk, and who subsequently underwent endovascular balloon angioplasty with stent placement reported favorable outcomes (although long-term follow-up was lacking).[58] Small vessel caliber and angulation of the vertebral vessels make endovascular treatment technically challenging. Generally, because of the high risk of complications, angioplasty of the basilar artery is advised only for patients with severe symptoms who have failed traditional medical therapy.[43] Randomized prospective trials of endovascular therapy are lacking.

Admission criteria

With few, if any, exceptions, all patients with PCS should be admitted to the hospital, preferably under the care of a stroke specialist. Patients may require intensive care unit level care if their stroke is of a large volume; if there is thought be a significant area of brain tissue at risk for further injury; if critical brainstem function is threatened; if they have received acute intervention, such as thrombolytics; or if they have significant comorbid medical conditions. Examinations aimed at identifying the cause of the stroke should be undertaken and risk-factor modification should be addressed.

SUMMARY

Dizzy patients present a significant diagnostic challenge to the emergency clinician. Discrimination between peripheral and central causes is important and will inform subsequent diagnostic evaluation and treatment. Isolated vertigo can be the only initial symptom of a PCS. The sensation of imbalance especially raises this possibility. Research involving strokes of the posterior circulation has lagged behind that of the anterior cerebral circulation. Investigations of the last 20 years, using new technologies in brain imaging in combination with detailed clinical studies, have revolutionized our understanding of the clinical presentation, causes, treatments, and prognosis of posterior circulation ischemia.[38] Traditional teaching, which emphasized differences in the cause, diagnosis, and treatment of ACS and PCS, must be reconsidered, and the entities may be more similar than initially thought. The approach to patients with PCS should be no different from those with strokes elsewhere in the brain: the immediate goals are to correctly identify stroke as a diagnostic possibility, determine the time of onset, proceed with rapid imaging, and involve neurologic expertise. The ED physician must maintain a high index of suspicion for PCS because patients may present in a more subtle fashion that those with ACS. Further research examining optimal medical and interventional therapy for patients with PCS is needed.

REFERENCES

1. Burt CW, Schappert SM. Ambulatory care visits to physician offices, hospital outpatient departments, and emergency departments: United States, 1999–2000. Vital Health Stat 13 2004;(157):1–70.
2. Kerber KA, Meurer WJ, West BT, et al. Dizziness presentations in U.S. emergency departments, 1995-2004. Acad Emerg Med 2008;15(8):744–50.

3. Froehling DA, Silverstein MD, Mohr DN, et al. Benign positional vertigo: incidence and prognosis in a population-based study in Olmsted County, Minnesota. Mayo Clin Proc 1991;66(6):596–601.
4. Sloane PD, Coeytaux RR, Beck RS, et al. Dizziness: state of the science. Ann Intern Med 2001;134(9 Pt 2):823–32.
5. Lawson J, Fitzgerald J, Birchall J, et al. Diagnosis of geriatric patients with severe dizziness. J Am Geriatr Soc 1999;47(1):12–7.
6. Baloh RW. Dizziness: neurological emergencies. Neurol Clin 1998;16(2):305–21.
7. Kerber KA, Brown DL, Lisabeth LD, et al. Stroke among patients with dizziness, vertigo, and imbalance in the emergency department: a population-based study. Stroke 2006;37(10):2484–7.
8. Eviatar L. Dizziness in children. Otolaryngol Clin North Am 1994;27(3):557–71.
9. Mallinson AI, Longridge NS. Dizziness from whiplash and head injury: differences between whiplash and head injury. Am J Otol 1998;19(6):814–8.
10. Marzo SJ, Leonetti JP, Raffin MJ, et al. Diagnosis and management of post-traumatic vertigo. Laryngoscope 2004;114(10):1720–3.
11. Young YH, Chen CH. Acute vertigo following cervical manipulation. Laryngoscope 2003;113(4):659–62.
12. Lee H, Sohn SI, Cho YW, et al. Cerebellar infarction presenting isolated vertigo: frequency and vascular topographical patterns. Neurology 2006;67(7): 1178–83.
13. Fife TD, Baloh RW, Duckwiler GR. Isolated dizziness in vertebrobasilar insufficiency: clinical features, angiography, and follow-up. J Stroke Cerebrovasc Dis 1994;4(1):4–12.
14. Son EJ, Bang JH, Kang JG. Anterior inferior cerebellar artery infarction presenting with sudden hearing loss and vertigo. Laryngoscope 2007;117(3):556–8.
15. Kim AS, Fullerton HJ, Johnston SC. Risk of vascular events in emergency department patients discharged home with diagnosis of dizziness or vertigo. Ann Emerg Med 2011;57(1):34–41.
16. Newman-Toker DE, Hsieh YH, Camargo CA Jr, et al. Spectrum of dizziness visits to US emergency departments: cross-sectional analysis from a nationally representative sample. Mayo Clin Proc 2008;83(7):765–75.
17. Newman-Toker DE. Charted records of dizzy patients suggest emergency physicians emphasize symptom quality in diagnostic assessment. Ann Emerg Med 2007;50(2):204–5.
18. Herr RD, Zun L, Mathews JJ. A directed approach to the dizzy patient. Ann Emerg Med 1989;18(6):664–72.
19. Gizzi M, Riley E, Molinari S. The diagnostic value of imaging the patient with dizziness. A Bayesian approach. Arch Neurol 1996;53(12):1299–304.
20. Johkura K, Momoo T, Kuroiwa Y. Positional nystagmus in patients with chronic dizziness. J Neurol Neurosurg Psychiatry 2008;79(12):1324–6.
21. De Marchis GM, Kohler A, Renz N, et al. Posterior versus anterior circulation strokes: comparison of clinical, radiological and outcome characteristics. J Neurol Neurosurg Psychiatry 2011;82(1):33–7.
22. Flossmann E, Rothwell PM. Prognosis of vertebrobasilar transient ischaemic attack and minor stroke. Brain 2003;126(Pt 9):1940–54.
23. Bogousslavsky J, Van Melle G, Regli F. The Lausanne Stroke Registry: analysis of 1,000 consecutive patients with first stroke. Stroke 1988;19(9):1083–92.
24. Caplan LR, Wityk RJ, Glass TA, et al. New England Medical Center Posterior Circulation registry. Ann Neurol 2004;56(3):389–98.
25. Becker KJ. Vertebrobasilar ischemia. New Horiz 1997;5(4):305–15.

26. Baumlin KM, Richardson LD. Stroke syndromes. Emerg Med Clin North Am 1997; 15(3):551–61.

27. Searls DE, Pazdera L, Korbel E, et al. Symptoms and signs of posterior circulation ischemia in the New England Medical Center Posterior Circulation Registry. Arch Neurol 2012;69(3):346–51.

28. Akhtar N, Kamran SI, Deleu D, et al. Ischaemic posterior circulation stroke in State of Qatar. Eur J Neurol 2009;16(9):1004–9.

29. Ferbert A, Bruckmann H, Drummen R. Clinical features of proven basilar artery occlusion. Stroke 1990;21(8):1135–42.

30. Gulli G, Khan S, Markus HS. Vertebrobasilar stenosis predicts high early recurrent stroke risk in posterior circulation stroke and TIA. Stroke 2009;40(8): 2732–7.

31. Bryan RN, Levy LM, Whitlow WD, et al. Diagnosis of acute cerebral infarction: comparison of CT and MR imaging. AJNR Am J Neuroradiol 1991;12(4):611–20.

32. Caplan L. Posterior circulation ischemia: then, now, and tomorrow. The Thomas Willis Lecture-2000. Stroke 2000;31(8):2011–23.

33. Linfante I, Llinas RH, Schlaug G, et al. Diffusion-weighted imaging and National Institutes of Health Stroke Scale in the acute phase of posterior-circulation stroke. Arch Neurol 2001;58(4):621–8.

34. Sato S, Toyoda K, Uehara T, et al. Baseline NIH Stroke Scale Score predicting outcome in anterior and posterior circulation strokes. Neurology 2008;70(24 Part 2):2371–7.

35. Kothari RU, Pancioli A, Liu T, et al. Cincinnati prehospital stroke scale: reproducibility and validity. Ann Emerg Med 1999;33(4):373–8.

36. Johnston SC, Rothwell PM, Nguyen-Huynh MN, et al. Validation and refinement of scores to predict very early stroke risk after transient ischaemic attack. Lancet 2007;369(9558):283–92.

37. Gulli G, Markus HS. The use of FAST and ABCD2 scores in posterior circulation, compared with anterior circulation, stroke and transient ischemic attack. J Neurol Neurosurg Psychiatry 2012;83(2):228–9.

38. Savitz SI, Caplan LR. Vertebrobasilar disease. N Engl J Med 2005;352(25): 2618–26.

39. Barnett HJ. A modern approach to posterior circulation ischemic stroke. Arch Neurol 2002;59(3):359–60.

40. Tsao JW, Hemphill JC 3rd, Johnston SC, et al. Initial Glasgow Coma Scale score predicts outcome following thrombolysis for posterior circulation stroke. Arch Neurol 2005;62(7):1126–9.

41. Furlan A, Higashida R, Wechsler L, et al. Intra-arterial prourokinase for acute ischemic stroke. The PROACT II study: a randomized controlled trial. Prolyse in acute cerebral thromboembolism. JAMA 1999;282(21):2003–11.

42. Tissue plasminogen activator for acute ischemic stroke. The National Institute of Neurological Disorders and Stroke rt-PA Stroke Study Group. N Engl J Med 1995; 333(24):1581–7.

43. Misra M, Alp M, Hier D, et al. Multidisciplinary treatment of posterior circulation ischemia. Neurol Res 2004;26(1):67–73.

44. Rothrock JF, Hart RG. Antithrombotic therapy in cerebrovascular disease. Ann Intern Med 1991;115(11):885.

45. Hass WK, Easton JD, Adams HP Jr, et al. A randomized trial comparing ticlopidine hydrochloride with aspirin for the prevention of stroke in high-risk patients. N Engl J Med 1989;321(8):501–7.

46. Farrell B, Godwin J, Richards S, et al. The United Kingdom transient ischaemic attack (UK-TIA) aspirin trial: final results. J Neurol Neurosurg Psychiatry 1991; 54(12):1044.

47. Grotta J, Norris J, Kamm B, et al. Prevention of stroke with ticlopidine. Neurology 1992;42(1):111–5.

48. Hacke W, Kaste M, Fieschi C, et al. Intravenous thrombolysis with recombinant tissue plasminogen activator for acute hemispheric stroke. The European Cooperative Acute Stroke Study (ECASS). JAMA 1995;274(13):1017–25.

49. Hacke W, Kaste M, Fieschi C, et al. Randomised double-blind placebo-controlled trial of thrombolytic therapy with intravenous alteplase in acute ischaemic stroke (ECASS II). Second European-Australasian Acute Stroke Study Investigators. Lancet 1998;352(9136):1245–51.

50. Clark WM, Wissman S, Albers GW, et al. Recombinant tissue-type plasminogen activator (Alteplase) for ischemic stroke 3 to 5 hours after symptom onset. The ATLANTIS Study: a randomized controlled trial. Alteplase Thrombolysis for Acute Noninterventional Therapy in Ischemic Stroke. JAMA 1999;282(21):2019–26.

51. Clark WM, Albers GW, Madden KP, et al. The rtPA (alteplase) 0- to 6-hour acute stroke trial, part A (A0276g): results of a double-blind, placebo-controlled, multicenter study. Thrombolytic therapy in acute ischemic stroke study investigators. Stroke 2000;31(4):811–6.

52. Hacke W, Kaste M, Bluhmki E, et al. Thrombolysis with alteplase 3 to 4.5 hours after acute ischemic stroke. N Engl J Med 2008;359(13):1317–29.

53. Grond M, Rudolf J, Schmulling S, et al. Early intravenous thrombolysis with recombinant tissue-type plasminogen activator in vertebrobasilar ischemic stroke. Arch Neurol 1998;55(4):466–9.

54. Montavont A, Nighoghossian N, Derex L, et al. Intravenous r-TPA in vertebrobasilar acute infarcts. Neurology 2004;62(10):1854–6.

55. Schonewille WJ, Wijman CA, Michel P, et al. Treatment and outcomes of acute basilar artery occlusion in the Basilar Artery International Cooperation Study (BASICS): a prospective registry study. Lancet Neurol 2009;8(8):724–30.

56. Lindsberg PJ, Soinne L, Tatlisumak T, et al. Long-term outcome after intravenous thrombolysis of basilar artery occlusion. JAMA 2004;292(15):1862–6.

57. Sarikaya H, Arnold M, Engelter ST, et al. Outcomes of intravenous thrombolysis in posterior versus anterior circulation stroke. Stroke 2011;42(9):2498–502.

58. Malek AM, Higashida RT, Phatouros CC, et al. Treatment of posterior circulation ischemia with extracranial percutaneous balloon angioplasty and stent placement. Stroke 1999;30(10):2073–85.

as a standard of care and includes both well-established medical therapies and emerging endovascular strategies.

The National Institute of Neurological Disorders and Stroke (NINDS) trial[2] in 1995 initiated the approval of intravenous (IV) recombinant tissue plasminogen activator (rt-PA) for AIS patients presenting within the 3-hour time window of symptom onset; treatment with IV rt-PA was extended to 4.5 hours by the European Cooperative Acute Stroke Study III study in 2008.[3] The efficacy of IV rt-PA has been limited, however, in large vessel occlusion due to lower recanalization rates, ranging from 10% for internal carotid artery (ICA) to 30% for proximal middle cerebral artery (MCA) occlusions.[4,5] Thrombus length in the MCA of greater than 8 mm was shown to have almost no chance of recanalization with rt-PA alone.[6] Persistence of ischemic penumbra beyond 3 hours of onset has been correlated with potentially salvageable brain tissue if adequate recanalization efforts are implemented.

Endovascular therapy to achieve recanalization using catheter-based approaches either includes intra-arterial thrombolysis (IAT) or mechanical endovascular therapy. This serves as an alternative treatment of AIS in patients who are either ineligible for IV thrombolysis (IVT) or present beyond the IVT time window. It is also an option for patients who do not improve after IVT. The advantage of IAT is that it allows direct delivery of a highly concentrated thrombolytic drug to the site of thrombus within the end-organ distribution and permits lower total dosage of systemic thrombolytics required to achieve recanalization. The other advantage is that mechanical thrombectomy may spare use of a pharmacologic thrombolytic entirely. The first US Food and Drug Administration (FDA) approval of endovascular therapy in acute stroke patients occurred in 2004 with the approval of Mechanical Embolus Removal in Cerebral Ischemia (MERCI) trial device to treat cerebral vessel occlusion.[7]

Endovascular therapy–based recanalization allows for direct clot disruption in a cerebral artery up to 8 hours from symptom onset in anterior circulation stroke and up to 12 hours from symptom onset in posterior circulation stroke. **Table 1** lists both currently accepted and investigational reperfusion strategies for AIS management. Among the available endovascular reperfusion strategies, the following are described in the literature (**Fig. 1**) and referenced in **Table 1**: recanalization or antegrade reperfusion, global reperfusion (flow augmentation or transarterial retrograde reperfusion), and transvenous retrograde reperfusion (flow reversal).[8,9]

The pathophysiology of AIS may have a thromboembolic origin (cardioembolic, large artery to artery embolism, intracranial atherosclerosis leading to thrombosis or hypoperfusion, vasculitis, and/or venous thrombosis) or hemodynamic mechanism. Thromboembolic strokes are managed pharmacologically or by an endovascular approach. Hemodynamic strokes can be managed medically with antithrombotic agents, statins, or permissive hypertension or managed surgically with carotid endarterectomy (CEA) or stenting. In medically refractory cases of hemodynamic stroke, angioplasty/stenting of extracranial or intracranial vessels or extracranial-intracranial bypass procedures may be considered as last resort to prevent progressive brain infarction.

IAT has been shown an alternative treatment of AIS in a selected patient population.[10–12] The current data are not adequate, however, for a conclusion to be drawn and require randomized controlled trials comparing endovascular therapy with IV rt-PA or best medical management. A phase III, randomized, multicenter open-label clinical trial, Interventional Management of Stroke (IMS) III,[13] to determine the efficacy of the combined IVT/IAT approach to treat acute stroke, was recently stopped after recruitment of 656 of a potential 900 patients because the primary outcome of the study, improvement in modified Rankin scale (mRS) at 3 months, met the threshold

Table 1
Currently available and investigational reperfusion strategies in acute stroke management

Recanalization or antegrade reperfusion approaches	IV and/or IAT	Thrombolytic agents: plasminogen activators, fibrinolytic agents
		Adjunctive therapy: heparin, direct thrombin inhibitors, glycoprotein IIb/IIIa antagonists
	Endovascular thrombectomy	Distal devices: MERCI, phenox, Solitaire, Trevo, Neuronet, Catch, Attracter-18
		Proximal devices: Alligator, In-Time Retriever, snares
	Endovascular thromboaspiration	Penumbra, AngioJet, F.A.S.T. Funnel Catheter
	Mechanical thrombus disruption	Microguidewire, snares, balloon angioplasty, Stent, OmniWave
	Transcranial or endovascular augmented fibrinolysis	TCD, EKOS, OmniWave
	Endovascular thrombus entrapment	Self-expanding and balloon-expandable stents
	Temporary endovascular bypass	Resheathable (closed-cell) stents, Solitaire, Trevo, ReVasc
Alternative reperfusion approaches	Global reperfusion (flow augmentation or transarterial retrograde reperfusion)	Pharmacologic: vasopressors (eg, phenylephrine)
		Mechanical: NeuroFlo
	Transvenous retrograde reperfusion (flow reversal)	Partial: retrograde transvenous neuroperfusion
		Complete: ReviveFlow

for futility. Patients in this trial were randomized to receive IVT alone or IVT/IAT in combination. Patients in the IVT/IAT arm of IMS III were only allowed to undergo one modality of intervention, whether it was intra-arterial (IA) rt-PA, MERCI, EKOS catheter, Penumbra, or Solitaire embolectomy.

In other case series, multimodal therapy has shown better recanalization rates in comparison with single therapy. The disadvantages to endovascular therapy include the complexity of the procedure, the level of required technical expertise, delays in initiating treatment, and the additional risks of an invasive procedure compared with IV rt-PA. Studies by Qureshi and colleagues[14] and Alexandrov and Grotta[12] showed early reocclusion in as many as 17% of patients treated with IAT and 34% of patients treated with IV rt-PA. Because multiple factors may be involved, no single specific

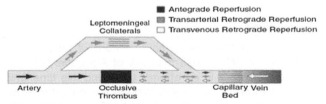

Fig. 1. Approaches to proposed modes of recanalization. (*Data from* Nogueira RG, Liebeskind DS, Sung G, et al, MERCI, Multi MERCI Writing Committee. Predictors of good clinical outcomes, mortality, and successful revascularization in patients with acute ischemic stroke undergoing thrombectomy: pooled analysis of the Mechanical Embolus Removal in Cerebral Ischemia [MERCI] and Multi MERCI Trials. Stroke 2009;40:3777–83.)

site of thrombosis. At present, no direct comparison trials have been reported between any of these agents. The choice, composition, and dose of agent are specific to each institution, with rt-PA (alteplase) the most frequently used agent in clinical practice. Recanalization rates for IAT have been shown superior to those for IVT for large vessel occlusions (ie, proximal MCA, carotid terminus, and basilar artery), averaging 70% versus 34%.[30–32]

Safety and efficacy of IA thrombolytic infusion using recombinant prourokinase–based therapy were established by the Prolyse in Acute Cerebral Thromboembolism (PROACT) I and II trials. PROACT I and II are multicenter randomized controlled trials (RCTs). In these studies, subjects with an MCA occlusion (baseline median NIHSS score of 17 and mean age of 66 years) were randomized to IA prourokinase and IV heparin or IA placebo with IV heparin initiated within 6 hours of stroke onset. The primary clinical outcome (mRS score ≤2) was achieved in 40% of the patients in the prourokinase treatment group compared with 25% in the control group (absolute benefit 15%; relative benefit 58%; number needed to treat = 7; $P = .043$). Although these trials presented encouraging data, the results of PROACT II were considered insufficient; hence, approval was not granted for the use of prourokinase in AIS. A larger RCT was recommended to establish the safety and efficacy of prourokinase but has not been initiated.

The Middle Cerebral Artery Embolism Local Fibrinolytic Intervention Trial (MELT) was another randomized trial that evaluated the safety and efficacy of IA urokinase in patients with MCA occlusions (M1 or M2) of fewer than 6 hours' duration.[33] IA urokinase infusion of 120,000 U was given for 5 minutes and repeated until the total dose reached 600,000 U; 2 hours had passed; or complete recanalization was achieved. This trial enrolled 114 patients and was stopped by the steering committee after the approval of IV rt-PA in Japan. The primary endpoint of mRS, less than or equal to 2, was not significantly different between the 57 patients in the treatment arm and 57 patients in the control arm (49.1% vs 38.6%; $P = .345$). Based on the results reported from the preplanned secondary analysis, the rate of recovery was normal or near normal (mRS ≤1) and was higher in the treatment group than in the controls (42.1% vs 22.8%; $P = .045$). The rate of ICH noticed was also similar to that seen in the PROACT II treatment patients (9%) and controls (2%).[33]

COMBINED IVT AND IAT

The Emergency Management of Stroke Bridging trial initiated in 1999 was one of the first trials performed to evaluate combined IVT and IAT. Thirty-five patients (mean age 65.6 years with a baseline mean NIHSS score of 16) with acute stroke were randomized to receive partial dose of IV rt-PA (0.6 mg/kg, 60 mg maximum) or placebo followed by IAT (mean dose 56.6 mg in the treatment arm vs 11.1 mg in the placebo arm) if the vessel remained occluded. Even though 70% of patients who received IV rt-PA still had angiographically confirmed residual thrombus requiring IAT, those who received the combination of IVT/IAT had significantly more MCA recanalization than the placebo group (55% vs 10%) with similar hemorrhagic complication rates. Clinical outcomes were comparable in these 2 groups.

A reversed bridging approach was proposed by Keris and colleagues,[34] in which 12 patients (mean age 53 years and mean NIHSS 25) with proximal vessel occlusions received IAT first with IV rt-PA administered afterward in an ICU (25 mg IA over 5–10 minutes followed by 60 minutes of 25-mg IV infusion). The control group included 33 patients who did not undergo any thrombolysis. There were no symptomatic ICHs (sICHs), and at 12 months, 83% of the patients in the thrombolysis group were functionally independent, whereas 33% of the control subjects had a good outcome. The mortality rates at 12 months were 17% and 64%, respectively.

The IMS trial[35] is the largest randomized controlled trial on bridging IVT to IAT and was first published in 2004. Eighty patients with a median baseline NIHSS score of 18 received IV rt-PA within 3 hours of onset followed by a 2-hour infusion of IA rt-PA (maximum dose 22 mg). Primary comparisons were conducted against a similar subset of placebo and IV rt-PA–treated patients from the NINDS rt-PA trial. The 3-month mortality rate of 16% was less than, but not statistically different from, the rate observed in the placebo (24%) and IV rt-PA treatment (21%) groups from the NINDS trial. The rate of sICH (6.3%) was similar to the rt-PA–treated group (6.6%) but higher than that in the placebo group (1%). The patients in the IMS trial had significantly better outcomes at 3 months (56%) than the NINDS placebo group for all outcome measures.

The IMS II trial[36] enrolled subjects age 18 to 80 years with a baseline NIHSS score greater than 10. Patients received IV-rtPA (0.6 mg/kg over 30 minutes) within 3 hours of symptom onset. For subjects with an arterial occlusion demonstrated at angiography, additional rt-PA was administered via the EKOS microinfusion catheter (EKOS Corporation, Bothell, Washington) or a standard microcatheter at the site of the thrombus up to a total dose of 22 mg over a 2-hour infusion time or until thrombolysis had been achieved. All IMS II subjects treated with IA rt-PA via microcatheter had a 60% (33/55) thrombolysis in cerebral infarction (TICI)/thrombolysis in myocardial infarction (TIMI) 2 and 3 reperfusion grade flow after completion of the IAT. The 3-month mortality in IMS II subjects was 16% and 46% of subjects had an mRS of 0 to 2.

The ongoing IMS III trial[13] is a phase III, randomized, multicenter, open-label clinical trial to determine the efficacy of the combined IVT/IAT approach to treat acute stroke. The patients are randomized to receive IV rt-PA alone or IVT/IAT combination. The patients in the IVT/IAT arm receive IV rt-PA and undergo immediate angiography. If an appropriate thrombus is identified, the neurointerventionalist may select either a standard or EKOS microcatheter to infuse rt-PA or select one of the mechanical devices, the MERCI retriever or Penumbra system, per user preference. The primary outcome measure is the rate of good clinical outcomes (mRS ≤2) at 90 days. The primary safety measure is mortality at 3 months and ICH within 24 hours of randomization. The trial initiated enrollment in 2006 and was stopped in April 2012 after enrollment of 656 of 900 subjects due to futility with respect to the primary outcome of mRS at 3 months. Further detail on the trial results is pending at this time.[37]

A meta-analysis by Georgiadis and colleagues[38] compared the use of partial with full-dose IV rt-PA followed by endovascular treatment and proposed that full-dose IVT is safe and may result in higher recanalization rates with better functional outcome at 3 months when combined with endovascular therapy. A retrospective analysis by Zaidat and colleagues[39] reviewed 96 patients (89 with occlusion in the anterior and 7 in the posterior circulation) who received IV and IA (n = 41) or IA rt-PA alone (n = 55). Among the 96 patients, 66 patients had any recanalization and 30 patients had no recanalization. A 19.7% mortality rate was reported at 90 days in the patients who had any recanalization whereas 33% mortality was reported in the group with no recanalization. Only 24% of the patients were reported to have achieved complete recanalization.

In a single institution, Recanalisation Using Combined Intravenous Alteplase and Neurointerventional Algorithm for Acute Ischemic Stroke (RECANALISE),[40] a prospective cohort study, was conducted to compare IVT with IVT followed by endovascular therapy approach: 107 patients were treated with IVT for large vessel occlusion compared with 53 patients treated with IVT followed by endovascular therapy.

feasibility of this device at 2 centers in United States. This device received approval based on the safety and efficacy data from studies in animal models to study laser treatment in 12 acute stroke patients. In this study, patients could receive treatment as late as 8 hours after symptom onset in the anterior circulation and within 24 hours in the posterior circulation. Difficulty with delivering the device to the clot location was the primary reason this trial was stopped.

Currently, another device in phase II trials being studied is an endovascular photo-acoustic recanalization (EPAR) laser system (EndoVasix, Belmont, California). This device is a mechanical clot fragmentation device in which photonic energy is con-verted to acoustic energy at the fiberoptic tip through creation of microcavitation bubbles. A pilot study showed overall recanalization rate of 41.1% (14/34) with a high mortality rate of 38.2%. There were 34 patients enrolled in this trial. **Table 2** lists all the randomized controlled trials on management of AIS, and **Table 3** lists the clin-ical trials using available mechanical devices for AIS management.

SONOTHROMBOLYSIS

Transcranial Doppler (TCD) color sonography is a procedure where B-mode imaging and pulsed Doppler sonography are combined to identify the target segment. Patients receive 1 hour of continuous monitoring and, once the Doppler sample volume is iden-tified, pulsed Doppler mode is applied. The operator must find the correct cerebral anatomy for successful application of this technique. Because the temporal bone has the minimal thickness when compared with the other bones of the cranium, use of the temporal region is considered a more successful approach for application of TCD.

To evaluate the safety and efficacy of TCD in management of AIS patients, several studies have been conducted. The Combined Lysis of Thrombus in Brain Ischemia using Transcranial Ultrasound and systemic TPA (CLOTBUST) study[49,50] was a multi-center RCT that enrolled 126 subjects treated with either TCD and IV rt-PA or IV rt-PA alone. Patients presenting with an occluded MCA within 3 hours of stroke onset were administered a standard IV rt-PA dose of 0.9 mg/kg. In the treatment group, TCD was administered simultaneously. Follow-up measurements of intracerebral blood flow were performed at 30, 60, 90, and 120 minutes after IV rt-PA bolus administration in both groups. If no early recanalization was observed, patients were immediately trans-ported to the angiography unit for IA intervention. Additional IAT with mechanical disruption of the thrombus was performed in 14% and 18% of patients in the target and control group. Sustained complete recanalization at 2 hours was achieved in

Table 2
Randomized controlled trials on acute ischemic stroke management

Baseline Characteristics	NINDS rt-PA	NINDS Control	PROACT II UK	PROACT II Control	MELT UK	MELT Control	SWIFT Solitaire
Patients (n)	312	312	121	59	57	57	113
Age (y)	68	66	64	64	67	67	67
Baseline NIHSS score	18	18	17	17	14	14	8–30
Revascularization %	—	—	66	18	73	—	83.3
sICH (%)	7	1	10.9	2	9	2	1.7
Asymptomatic ICH (%)	—	—	24	—	—	—	—
90-d mortality (%)	24	21	25	27	5.3	3.5	17.2
90-d mRS <2 (%)	28	30	40	25	49.1	38.6	—

Table 3 Major clinical trials of mechanical devices used for management of acute ischemic stroke				
Baseline Characteristics	MERCI Pilot	MERCI I	Multi MERCI	PENUMBRA
N	28	151	164	125
Age (mean)	68	67	68	64
NIHSS (mean)	22	20	19	18
Time to treatment (h)	2.5	4.3	4.3	4.3
Recanalization (TIMI 2–3) (%)	43	46	57	82
Hemorrhage (sICH) (%)	43	7.8	9.8	28
Outcome (mRS 0–2) at 90 d (%)		28	36	25

Data from Meyers PM, Schumacher HC, Connolly ES Jr, et al. Current status of endovascular stroke treatment. Circulation 2011;123(22):2591–601.

38% of patients in the target group compared with 13% in the control group; 42% of the target group and 29% of the control patient population had a favorable clinical outcome with mRS of 0–1. The 90-day mortality rates of 15% and 18% were observed for the target and control groups, respectively.

A prospective, nonrandomized, multicenter, phase II clinical study, Transcranial Low-Frequency Ultrasound-Mediated Thrombolysis in Brain Ischemia (TRUMBI), conducted to evaluate the safety and efficacy of sonothrombolysis, was stopped prematurely due to a significant increase in ICH rate in the target group.

ANGIOPLASTY OR STENT PLACEMENT

Over time, the feasibility and efficacy of percutaneous transluminal angioplasty (PTA) in acute stroke was demonstrated by various clinical studies. The balloon was initially used as a rescue procedure to displace thrombus or after early re-occlusion after successful fibrinolysis. Angioplasty followed by stenting was described in acute stroke management for underlying atherosclerotic stenosis after successful fibrinolysis. Recanalization postangioplasty is successful with high rates (60%–90%) with or without accompanying fibrinolysis.

Nakano and colleagues[50] conducted one of the largest studies demonstrating the efficacy and usefulness of PTA in 36 patients who presented with acute strokes and underwent thrombolytic therapy (IV or IA) alone compared with 34 patients who were treated first with PTA and subsequent thrombolytic therapy as needed for distal embolization. Partial or complete recanalization was achieved in 63.9% versus 91.2% in the combined group. sICH was seen in 19.4% versus 2.9%, and good outcome (mRS ≤2) occurred in 50% versus 73.5% of patients. Risk of rethrombosis may be higher in patients with atherothrombotic disease due to restenosis. In patients in whom cerebral blood flow cannot be maintained by medical therapy, PTA may be used as a salvage technique. Low-pressure, more-compliant balloons are used to improve the safety of this procedure.

Development of self-expanding stents has been another modality for the treatment of AIS. The first prospective FDA-approved trial, Stent-Assisted Recanalization in Acute Ischemic Stroke,[51] demonstrated 100% recanalization in 20 patients. There was 1 (5%) sICH, and 1-month mRS was 0 or 1 in 45% of the treated patients. The disadvantage of this approach, however, lies with the implantation of a permanent vascular prosthesis and the necessity of dual antiplatelet therapy initially after the procedure for 1 to 3 months, followed by indefinite single antiplatelet therapy.

Levy and colleagues[51] reported potential advantages of stent technology for AIS: it may provide both higher rates of recanalization and more rapid recanalization. Stents may be of particular interest in patients with underlying intracranial atherosclerotic lesions or focal recalcitrant clots. The majority of patients in the reported study underwent intracranial stent placement after failure of other treatment modalities. The recanalization rate was 78% in the 138 patients treated with intracranial stents with minimal hemorrhagic adverse events. Natarajan and colleagues[52] also reported on a retrospective series in which balloon-mounted stents were used in 19 patients. Stenting was performed as a last resort once other modes of treatment had failed to recanalize occluded arteries. An overall TIMI score of 2 or 3 was achieved in 79% of patients.

NEUROSURGICAL MANAGEMENT
Extracranial-Intracranial Bypass

Historically, bypass surgery was performed for patients presenting with strokes of hemodynamic origin rather than thromboembolic mechanisms. Superficial temporal artery to MCA bypass was introduced by Donaghy and Yasargil[53] in 1969, initiating the practice of bypass surgery. Extracranial-intracranial (EC-IC) bypass revascularizes ischemic brain by redirecting blood flow from the scalp through this low-flow surgical conduit. High-flow bypass uses saphenous vein grafts or radial artery grafts to connect cervical carotid donor arteries with intracranial recipient arteries and this eventually led to the development of bypass surgery. Although bypass techniques are applicable to complex aneurysms whose treatment might require deliberate occlusion of an afferent or efferent artery, these techniques are not as applicable to ischemic strokes because few are hemodynamic in origin.

In the past, bypass surgery was used for patients with atheroocclusive disease responsible for patients with chronic, low cerebral blood flow and intermittent episodes of ischemic symptoms. Symptoms of hemodynamic insufficiency due to atheroocclusive disease include transient ischemic attack or stroke, often provoked in the setting of hypotension or orthostatic intolerance. Intervention with bypass surgery was considered in patients with these 5 distinct conditions:

1. Extracranial atherosclerotic occlusive disease (ie, ICA occlusion)
2. Intracranial atherosclerotic steno-occlusive disease (ie, MCA occlusion and, rarely, high-grade MCA stenosis)
3. Vertebrobasilar atherosclerotic steno-occlusive disease
4. Vasculitis resulting in severe occlusive disease
5. Moyamoya disease

Traditionally, contraindications to bypass surgery were a large stroke on CT or MRI involving the entire territory of the affected artery, because this tissue is not salvageable and because revascularization may precipitate hemorrhagic conversion of an acute infarction.

Watershed infarcts that occur in the areas between vascular territories, such as between MCA and anterior cerebral artery (ACA) territories or between MCA and posterior cerebral artery (PCA) territories, are commonly seen in patients with atheroocclusive disease and hemodynamic insufficiency. Internal watershed infarcts at gray–white matter junction between superficial and deep perforators of the MCA are more suggestive of hemodynamic insufficiency than cortical watershed infarcts.

In cases where the traditional bypass arteries are not available, alternative bypass surgery with interposition grafts, like saphenous vein or radial artery with higher flow, can be performed. The cervical carotid artery is an accessible donor artery, with anastomotic sites on the ICA, ECA, and common carotid artery (CCA). The ICA is used in bypass when a patent stump is available and collateral circulation from the ECA must be preserved. ECA is used when the cerebral circulation is critically dependent on ICA flow and temporary ICA or CCA occlusion during the anastomosis would be poorly tolerated. The CCA is used when the carotid bifurcation is high riding and exposure is compromised by the mandible. High-flow bypasses connect the ICA, ECA, or CCA with the MCA, typically along the M2 segment distal to the lenticulostriate arteries originating from the M1 segment. Based on the randomized studies, the safety and efficacy of bypass surgery for the prevention of ischemic stroke have been unfavorable.

Randomized Controlled Trials

The multicenter EC-IC Bypass Trial[54] randomized 1377 patients to surgical or medical therapy and found no significant difference in stroke rates in surgical and medical patients (31% and 29%, respectively).

The Carotid Occlusion Surgery Study[55] used positron emission tomography and oxygen extraction factor to identify patients with hemodynamic insufficiency and examine the protective effect of bypass surgery. This prospective, randomized, multicenter trial was prematurely stopped because the interim analysis failed to demonstrate a difference between surgical and medical groups.

Carotid Endarterectomy

Emergency CEA for acute or progressive stroke is controversial. The potential benefit of emergency CEA was shown with patients with fluctuating neurologic deficit or progressive stroke with a satisfactory outcome (no or mild neurologic deficit) in as many as 84% of cases with an overall mortality rate of 6% to 20%. Prognostic factors to consider in these patients are timing of surgery, absence of cerebral coma, quality of collateral blood flow, and coexistence of simultaneous arterio-arterial embolization in the MCA. In patients who sustain a profound neurologic deficit caused by an acute extracranial carotid occlusion and underwent CEA, a stroke rate varying from 40% to 69% and mortality rate ranging from 16% to 55% have been observed. Comparable mortality in patients with intracranial ICA occlusion, occlusion of the MCA, or both is as high as 53%.

As reported by Eckstein and colleagues[56] in a nonrandomized pilot clinical study, 12 of 14 patients had the clinical signs of a major ischemic carotid-related stroke either caused by acute carotid occlusion in 9 of 12 patients or occlusions of the MCA (main stem and major branches, respectively). The 2 remaining patients sustained intracerebral embolism during elective CEA.

The 14 patients reported in this clinical study represent the first consecutive series in a single-center experience. Four patients recovered completely (mRS = 0), 6 had a minor stroke (mRS = 2–3), 2 had a major stroke (mRS = 4–5), and 2 patients died postoperatively. After 6 months, 7 patients were functionally independent (mRS = 0–1), 4 patients still had a mild or moderate deficit (mRS = 2–3), and 1 patient still had a severe deficit (mRS = 5). Because hemorrhagic transformation of an ischemic cerebral infarction occurred in 1 patient, the investigators did not report intraparenchymal hematoma.

Simultaneous occlusion of the MCA is another important factor for determining prognosis after emergent CEA. Meyer and colleagues[57] operated on 34 patients with profound neurologic deficits caused by acute carotid occlusions and achieved a good outcome in 38.3%, fair outcome in 29.4%, poor outcome in 11.8%, and death in 20.5%. Coexistence of MCA embolism strongly influenced patient recovery because 7 of 9 patients with MCA occlusions had a poor outcome or died. It was

23. del Zoppo GJ, Higashida RT, Furlan AJ, et al. PROACT: a phase II randomized trial of recombinant pro-urokinase by direct arterial delivery in acute middle cerebral artery stroke. PROACT Investigators. Prolyse in Acute Cerebral Thromboembolism. Stroke 1998;29(1):4–11.

24. Furlan A, Higashida R, Wechsler L, et al. Intra-arterial prourokinase for acute ischemic stroke. The PROACT II study: a randomized controlled trial. Prolyse in Acute Cerebral Thromboembolism. JAMA 1999;282(21):2003–11.

25. Ernst R, Pancioli A, Tomsick T, et al. Combined intravenous and intra-arterial recombinant tissue plasminogen activator in acute ischemic stroke. Stroke 2000; 31(11):2552–7.

26. Lewandowski CA, Frankel M, Tomsick TA, et al. Combined intravenous and intra-arterial r-TPA versus intra-arterial therapy of acute ischemic stroke: Emergency Management of Stroke (EMS) Bridging Trial. Stroke 1999;30(12):2598–605.

27. Suarez JI, Zaidat OO, Sunshine JL, et al. Endovascular administration after intravenous infusion of thrombolytic agents for the treatment of patients with acute ischemic strokes. Neurosurgery 2002;50(2):251–9 [discussion: 259–60].

28. Wolfe T, Suarez JI, Tarr RW, et al. Comparison of combined venous and arterial thrombolysis with primary arterial therapy using recombinant tissue plasminogen activator in acute ischemic stroke. J Stroke Cerebrovasc Dis 2008;17(3):121–8.

29. Moskowitz M, Caplan L. Thrombolytic treatment in acute stroke: review and update of selective topics. Cerebrovascular Diseases: Nineteenth Princeton Stroke Conference. Boston: Butterworth-Heinemann; 1995.

30. del Zoppo GJ, Ferbert A, Otis S, et al. Local intra-arterial fibrinolytic therapy in acute carotid territory stroke. A pilot study. Stroke 1988;19:307–13.

31. del Zoppo GJ, Poeck K, Pessin MS, et al. Recombinant tissue plasminogen activator in acute thrombotic and embolic stroke. Ann Neurol 1992;32:78–86.

32. Mattle HP, Arnold M, Georgiadis D, et al. Comparison of intraarterial and intravenous thrombolysis for ischemic stroke with hyperdense middle cerebral artery sign. Stroke 2008;39(2):379–83 [Epub 2007 Dec 20].

33. Ogawa A, Mori E, Minematsu K, et al. Randomized trial of intraarterial infusion of urokinase within 6 h of middle cerebral artery stroke: the middle cerebral artery embolism local fibrinolytic intervention trial (MELT) Japan. Stroke 2007;38:2633–9.

34. Keris V, Rudnicka S, Vorona V, et al. Combined intraarterial/intravenous thrombolysis for acute ischemic stroke. AJNR Am J Neuroradiol 2001;22(2):352–8.

35. IMS Study Investigators. Combined intravenous and intra-arterial recanalization for acute ischemic stroke: the Interventional Management of Stroke Study. Stroke 2004;35(4):904–11.

36. IMS II Trial Investigators. The Interventional Management of Stroke (IMS) II Study. Stroke 2007;38(7):2127–35.

37. Available at: http://clinicaltrials.gov/ct2/show/NCT00359424. Accessed May 11, 2012.

38. Georgiadis AL, Memon MZ, Shah QA, et al. Comparison of partial (.6 mg/kg) versus full-dose (.9 mg/kg) intravenous recombinant tissue plasminogen activator followed by endovascular treatment for acute ischemic stroke: a meta-analysis. J Neuroimaging 2011;21(2):113–20.

39. Zaidat OO, Suarez JI, Sunshine JL, et al. Thrombolytic therapy of acute ischemic stroke: correlation of angiographic recanalization with clinical outcome. AJNR Am J Neuroradiol 2005;26(4):880–4.

40. Mazighi M, Serfaty JM, Labreuche J, et al. Comparison of intravenous alteplase with a combined intravenous-endovascular approach in patients with stroke and confirmed arterial occlusion (RECANALISE study): a prospective cohort study. Lancet Neurol 2009;8:802–9.

41. Smith WS. Safety of mechanical thrombectomy and intravenous tissue plasminogen activator in acute ischemic stroke. Results of the multi Mechanical Embolus Removal in Cerebral Ischemia (MERCI) trial, part I. AJNR Am J Neuroradiol 2006; 27(6):1177–82.

42. Smith WS, Sung G, Saver J, et al, Multi MERCI Investigators. Mechanical thrombectomy for acute ischemic stroke: final results of the Multi MERCI trial. Stroke 2008;39(4):1205–12.

43. Josephson SA, Saver JL, Smith WS, MERCI and Multi MERCI Investigators. Comparison of mechanical embolectomy and intraarterial thrombolysis in acute ischemic stroke within the MCA: MERCI and Multi MERCI compared to PROACT II. Neurocrit Care 2009;10(1):43–9.

44. Seifert M, Ahlbrecht A, Dohmen C, et al. Combined interventional stroke therapy using intracranial stent and local intraarterial thrombolysis (LIT). Neuroradiology 2010;53:273–82.

45. Solitaire FR with the Intention for Thrombectomy (SWIFT). Available at: http:// clinicaltrials.gov/ct2/show/NCT01054560. Accessed May 11, 2012.

46. Penumbra Pivotal Stroke Trial Investigators. The penumbra pivotal stroke trial: safety and effectiveness of a new generation of mechanical devices for clot removal in intracranial large vessel occlusive disease. Stroke 2009;40(8):2761–8.

47. Gounis MJ, DeLeo MJ III, Wakhloo AK. Advances in interventional neuroradiology. Stroke 2010;41(2):e81–7.

48. Liebig T, Reinartz J, Guethe T, et al. Early clinical experiences with a new thrombectomy device for the treatment of ischemic stroke [abstract]. Stroke 2008;39: 608.

49. Alexandrov AV, Wojner AW, Grotta JC, CLOTBUST Investigators. CLOTBUST: design of a randomized trial of ultrasound-enhanced thrombolysis for acute ischemic stroke. J Neuroimaging 2004;14(2):108–12.

50. Nakano S, Iseda T, Yoneyama T, et al. Direct percutaneous transluminal angioplasty for acute middle cerebral artery trunk occlusion: an alternative option to intra-arterial thrombolysis. Stroke 2002;33(12):2872–6.

51. Levy EI, Siddiqui AH, Crumlish A, et al. First Food and Drug Administration-approved prospective trial of primary intracranial stenting for acute stroke: SARIS (stent-assisted recanalization in acute ischemic stroke). Stroke 2009;40(11): 3552–6.

52. Natarajan SK, Ogilvy CS, Hopkins LN, et al. Initial experience with an everolimus-eluting, second-generation drug-eluting stent for treatment of intracranial atherosclerosis. J Neurointerv Surg 2010;2(2):104–9.

53. Donaghy RM, Yasargil G. Microangeional surgery and its techniques. Prog Brain Res 1968;30:263–7.

54. Garrett MC, Komotar RJ, Merkow MB, et al. The extracranial-intracranial bypass trial: implications for future investigations. Neurosurg Focus 2008;24(2):E4.

55. Powers WJ, Clarke WR, Grubb RL Jr, et al, COSS Investigators. Extracranial-intracranial bypass surgery for stroke prevention in hemodynamic cerebral ischemia: the Carotid Occlusion Surgery Study randomized trial. JAMA 2011;306(18): 1983–92.

56. Eckstein HH, Schumacher H, Dörfler A, et al. Carotid endarterectomy and intracranial thrombolysis: simultaneous and staged procedures in ischemic stroke. J Vasc Surg 1999;29(3):459–71.

57. Meyer FB, Sundt TM Jr, Piepgras DG, et al. Emergency carotid endarterectomy for patients with acute carotid occlusion and profound neurological deficits. Ann Surg 1986;203(1):82–9.

further neuronal death through progressive infarction and secondary injury mechanisms. The goal of neurocritical care for the patient with acute ischemic stroke (AIS) is to optimize long-term functional outcomes and quality of life by minimizing the amount of brain tissue that is lost to these processes. This is accomplished by optimizing brain perfusion, limiting secondary brain injury, and compensating for associated dysfunction in other organ systems. Because of the rapid and irreversible nature of ischemic brain injury, it is crucial for best neurocritical care practices to begin as early as possible. Given data indicating that acute stroke patients might spend an average of 5 hours in the emergency department (ED),[4] it is clear that optimal neurocritical care should begin in the ED and not be delayed until the patient arrives in the intensive care unit (ICU). This article will discuss optimal, pragmatic neurocritical care management of patients with AIS during the golden ED hours from the perspective of the neurointensivist.

PRELIMINARY CONSIDERATIONS
Triage

Determination of what constitutes critical illness in the AIS patient can be challenging. AIS patients have markers of the need for critical care that are unique to AIS in the absence of the more typical signs of respiratory or hemodynamic instability. Chief among these is the potential for neurologic decline, which can be caused by progression of the initial stroke, early recurrent stroke in a different vascular territory, progressive cerebral edema with tissue shifts, and severe reperfusion injury.[5] Early in the course of evaluation of a patient with AIS, it can be difficult to accurately gauge an individual patient's risk for neurologic decline. At the same time, compared with other organs, the brain is exquisitely sensitive to ischemia and other physiologic perturbations; once injured, the adult brain heals very poorly. For these reasons, reactive management strategies are far less effective in patients with critical brain injuries than in illness primarily involving other organ systems. Optimal care for AIS patients, therefore, requires a hypervigilant strategy of prevention, early detection, and ultrarapid treatment of neurologic decline. It follows that all AIS patients should be considered to be critically ill, at least while they remain in the ED.

Physiologic Monitoring

Cardiovascular monitoring and respiratory monitoring in AIS do not differ significantly from that required for any other critically ill patient in the ED. Continuous cardiac telemetry and blood pressure monitoring every 5 to 10 minutes with an automated cuff are sufficient in most patients. In patients who require continuous antihypertensive or vasopressor infusions, an arterial catheter is the preferred method of blood pressure monitoring. Pulse oximetry and quantification of the respiratory rate are sufficient for most patients. However, due to the rapidity by which hypercapnia can develop and critically worsen cerebral edema and intracranial pressure (ICP), there should be a low threshold for the determination of the arterial partial pressure of carbon dioxide (CO_2) by arterial blood gas. Similarly, intubated AIS patients in the ED should ideally have the end–tidal CO_2 continuously monitored.

Several devices are currently available for continuous monitoring of key parameters of cerebral physiology beyond ICP, including brain tissue oxygen tension, cerebral blood flow, and electrical activity.[6] Cerebral microdialysis allows for the monitoring of the concentration of numerous small molecules in the hemispheric interstitium, giving a very precise picture of neuronal metabolic milieu.[7] Most of these devices are invasive, introduced into the brain through a small burr hole craniotomy in a fashion identical to the technique used to place the more familiar fiberoptic Camino ICP moni-tors (Integra LifeSciences, Plainsboro, New Jersey) and external ventricular drains. Despite solid physiologic underpinnings and early evidence of clinical utility, these devices have a number of limitations precluding their widespread use in contemporary clinical practice, especially in the ED setting. These include the time and expertise necessary to place the devices and interpret their results, the small associated risks of hemorrhage and infection, the relatively small volume of brain tissue that can be monitored, and, with the exception of intracranial and cerebral perfusion pressure, a lack of evidence that clearly supports benefit to the patient.

The neurologic examination, therefore, remains the most important tool for moni-toring the nervous system in patients with AIS. As with other physiologic parameters, serial measurements using a validated, reproducible, and easy technique provide the most valuable information. This can be accomplished by examining the patient every 15 minutes using the National Institutes of Health (NIH) Stroke Scale (NIHSS), which is essentially an efficient, abbreviated neurologic examination focused on the most salient features in stroke patients. An increase by 2 or more points on the NIHSS can generally be used as a threshold for clinically significant neurologic decline that should trigger repeat imaging of the brain and relevant vessels.[8]

The NIHSS is of limited utility for patients with more than mildly diminished arousal, who are more appropriately assessed with the use of a clinical scale specifically designed for coma. The Glasgow Coma Scale (GCS) has a significant floor phenom-enon, providing little useful neurologic information about patients with the lowest levels of consciousness. The Full Outline of UnResponsiveness (FOUR Score),[9] which incorporates more detailed testing of brainstem functions and assesses receptive rather than expressive language (as tested by the GCS), is a superior clinical assess-ment scale for comatose patients with AIS (**Fig. 1**). It is only slightly more complicated to learn and perform than the GCS, and it has been shown to be valid and reliable when performed in the ED by emergency physicians and nurses and in AIS patients.[10–12] A decline of 1 point on the FOUR Score should be considered clinically significant and trigger repeat imaging of the brain and relevant vessels.

CEREBRAL PERFUSION OPTIMIZATION

Few AIS patients undergo an acute reperfusion therapy.[3] Most AIS patients, therefore, are dependent on less direct measures of perfusion optimization to protect at-risk brain from progressing to infarction. These measures form the foundation of neurocrit-ical care for AIS and consist of careful blood pressure management with a preference for higher pressures, intravascular volume augmentation, and keeping the patient's head of bed low.

Treatment of Hypertension

The guiding principle of hemodynamic management for AIS patients in the first 24 hours after onset is that, in general, higher blood pressures are better than lower blood pressures.[2] Two pathophysiologic issues underlie this approach. First, to reach the ischemic penumbra, blood must either flow through the significant stenosis in the native circulation that is causing the stroke or travel through probably higher-resistance collateral routes in the case of occlusion of the native artery. Second, autor-egulation in ischemic brain is impaired, thus making flow (and therefore oxygen delivery) entirely dependent on perfusion pressure.[13] It is not surprising then, that both very high and very low initial blood pressures are associated with poor outcomes in AIS.[2,14] Most notably, a substantial body of evidence from clinical trials and

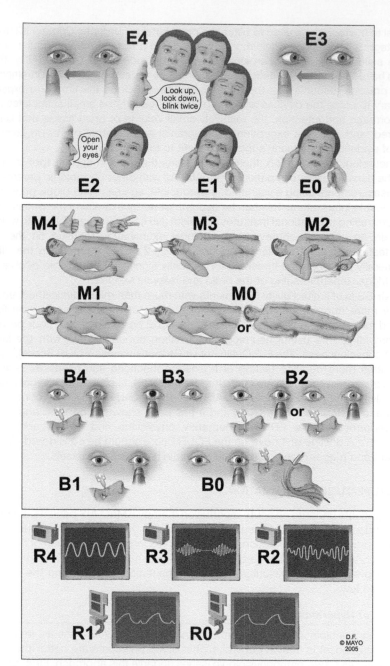

Fig. 1. The Full Outline of UnResponsiveness (FOUR) score. Four components of neurologic function are assessed: eye response (E), motor response (M), brainstem reflexes (B), and respiration (R). Each component is graded 0 to 4, with lower scores indicating more severe brain dysfunction. Instructions for using the scale can be found in the following reference. (*Reproduced from* Wijdicks EFM, Bamlet WR, Maramattom BV, et al. Validation of a new coma scale: the FOUR score. Ann Neurol 2005;58:585–93, by permission of Mayo Foundation for Medical Education and Research. All rights reserved.)

observational studies indicates that actively lowering the blood pressure in AIS patients in the first hours after onset is associated with acute neurologic deterioration and worse clinical outcomes.[14–17]

Based on this information, the most recent American Heart Association/American Stroke Association (AHA/ASA) guidelines for the treatment of AIS recommend a strategy of permissive hypertension. The blood pressure is allowed to rise to as high as 220/120 mm Hg before treatment is started unless the patient develops signs of end organ dysfunction due to hypertension (myocardial ischemia, congestive heart failure [CHF], renal failure, cerebral edema, intracerebral hemorrhage [ICH], retinal injury), in which case the blood pressure should be lowered to the highest level that is safely tolerated by the injured organ (a mean arterial pressure [MAP] reduction of about 10% to 20% of maximum for most patients).[2] For patients who have received intravenous rt-PA, the blood pressure must be kept strictly below 180/105 mm Hg in the first 24 hours after treatment to minimize the risk of ICH.[2]

Defining a target blood pressure for patients who have undergone acute endovascular revascularization is a difficult, empiric process that is different for each patient and for which there are no published data available for guidance. It is crucial to determine the goal blood pressure jointly with the endovascular specialist. Due to the empiric nature of determining a target blood pressure in these patients, meticulous attention must be paid to monitoring for signs of cerebral hypoperfusion (new or worsening deficits referable to the territory of the original stroke) and cerebral hyperperfusion (similar to hypoperfusion, but in addition headache, visual blurring, depressed arousal, and seizures).[18] Although treatment must be individualized for each patient, the authors' general blood pressure targets in hypertensive AIS patients are found in **Table 1**. **Box 1** summarizes their approach to acute antihypertensive management in AIS.[13,14,19]

Induced Hypertension

There is no strong evidence to support the use of induced hypertension in any population of AIS patients. However, case reports, case series, and 2 very small prospective studies provide preliminary evidence of safety and effectiveness when induced hypertension is applied carefully in highly selected patients. Markers of potential responsiveness to induced hypertension are listed in **Box 2**.[20]

The authors begin hemodynamic augmentation with augmentation of intravascular volume. Determining the optimal blood pressure is empiric. The authors typically raise the mean arterial pressure by 10% to 20% and then reassess 15 to 20 minutes later. If insufficient neurologic improvement has occurred, and the patient is tolerating the treatment, the authors will raise it by another 10%, to a maximum systolic blood

Table 1
Blood pressure targets when treating hypertension in AIS

Clinical Scenario	Blood Pressure Trigger for Treatment	Target Blood Pressure with Treatment
No end-organ dysfunction, no rt-PA	>220/110 mm Hg	SBP 180–200 mm Hg
First 24 h after rt-PA	180/105 mm Hg	SBP 155–175 mm Hg
Evidence of end-organ dysfunction	NA	Reduce MAP by 10%–20% and reassess
Postendovascular therapy	Individualized (see text)	Individualized (see text)

Abbreviation: SBP, systolic blood pressure.

displaces surrounding tissue, leading to horizontal displacement of the falx cerebri and horizontal and caudal shift of the thalamus and midbrain (**Fig. 2**). Clinical manifestations of these tissue shifts are listed in **Table 2**.[27] **Box 3** lists markers of increased risk for development of the malignant MCA syndrome.[30,32,33]

Mortality and morbidity in the malignant MCA syndrome are substantial. When treated with aggressive critical care—but without decompressive surgery—mortality is between 55% and 80%, and a large proportion of survivors have substantial neurologic deficits.[29,34,35] The first priorities of critical care management for patients at risk of developing this syndrome are prevention and early detection. Minimization of cerebral edema involves careful management of sedation and analgesia, fluid status, body temperature, and blood glucose. The patient's HOB should be elevated to 30°. If signs of herniation develop, the authors employ a step-wise medical management algorithm (**Box 4**).[36,37]

In the ED setting, the choice between mannitol and hypertonic saline is largely settled by which agent can be administered more quickly to the patient. Mannitol is more widely available, more familiar, and can be safely given through peripheral veins. It ultimately depletes intravascular volume through its diuretic effects, however, in contrast with hypertonic saline's potent volume-augmenting effects. Thus, hypertonic saline is preferred in patients who have intravascular volume depletion. Regarding the primary effect of lowering ICP, insufficient data exist to validly compare the effects of mannitol and hypertonic saline in the setting of AIS. A recent meta-analysis of 5 trials that compared the effect of equiosmolar doses of these agents in patients with mostly traumatic brain injury suggests that hypertonic saline may be somewhat more effective, but these are not conclusive data.[38]

Because medical treatment frequently fails to control edema and reverse or arrest tissue shift in large MCA infarcts, decompressive hemicraniectomy should be considered as soon as a patient manifests any signs of malignant edema. This treatment has recently been studied in 3 European randomized, prospective studies that included patients 18 to 60 years old.[35,39,40] Meta-analysis of pooled data from these studies indicates that, when performed within 48 hours of stroke onset, hemicraniectomy decreases 12-month mortality by about 50%.[35] This effect does not differ if the infarct is in the dominant or nondominant hemisphere. The gain in survival, unfortunately,

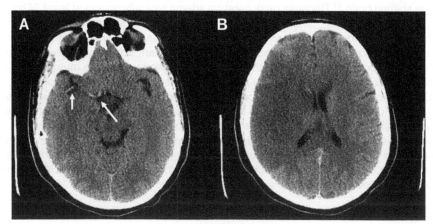

Fig. 2. CT images of a massive middle cerebral artery (MCA) infarction demonstrating the hyperdense MCA sign (*A, arrows*) and hypodensity in greater than 50% of the MCA territory (*B*).

Table 2	
Clinical manifestations of brain tissue shift and herniation in the malignant MCA syndrome	
Clinical Manifestation	**Anatomic Substrate**
Progressive decline in arousal	Displacement of the ascending reticular activating system in the midbrain and thalamus
Upgoing toe, then frank weakness on the side of the body ipsilateral to the infarct	Compression of the cerebral peduncle contralateral to the infarct against the adjacent edge of the tentorium; Kernohan notch phenomenon
Unilateral dilated, poorly reactive pupil	Compression or torquing of the third nerve as the midbrain shifts
Extensor posturing	Midbrain compression or shift

comes at the expense of a significant likelihood of surviving with severe disability; in the same meta-analysis, there was no significant effect of hemicraniectomy on reducing the proportion of patients with the combined outcome of death or severe disability.[35] Given these limitations, the authors typically offer decompressive hemicraniectomy only to patients 60 years old and younger who are in generally good health and who have no significant neurologic disability before the stroke. They are careful to inform surrogate decision makers that the goal of the operation is to increase the likelihood of survival and not necessarily to improve functional outcome, which may well be poor. Due to the lack of clear benefit when performed more than 48 hours after stroke onset,[35] the authors involve the neurosurgery team early in patients at risk for malignant MCA syndrome to facilitate operation at the earliest indication.

Massive Cerebellar Infarction

The posterior fossa contains little excess space to accommodate the additional mass of a swelling cerebellar infarct, to which the vital structures of the brainstem lie in close proximity (**Fig. 3**). Significant neurologic deterioration, therefore, is both common and can be rapidly fatal in patients with large infarctions of the cerebellum. These consequences occur by 2 main mechanisms of mass effect, which often develop in parallel:

- Obstructive hydrocephalus caused by compression of the fourth ventricle and its outlet foramina
- Direct compression of the brainstem, most typically the pontine tegmentum

Deterioration due to brainstem compression and hydrocephalus occurs in about 10% to 25% of patients with cerebellar infarction.[41–44] This decline most often occurs

Box 3
Markers of increased risk for the malignant MCA syndrome

- Clinical: NIHSS greater than 15
- Computed tomography (CT) scan:
  - Hypodensity in greater than 50% of the MCA territory
  - Hyperdense MCA sign
  - 2 of the following 3 signs: hypodense basal ganglia, hypodense insular ribbon, and effacement of hemispheric sulci

---

Box 4
Medical management of cerebral herniation

- Seek and treat easily reversible causes of elevated ICP (pain, agitation, seizure, blood pressure too high or too low, inadequate oxygenation and ventilation)
- Osmotherapy
  - Mannitol
    - Initial dose 1–1.5 g/kg intravenously
    - Subsequent doses 0.25–1 g/kg intravenously
    - Administer via peripheral or central vein over 10 to 20 minutes
    - Replace intravascular volume lost through diuresis with normal saline to avoid hypotension and kidney injury
    - Monitor electrolytes and serum osmolality
      - Do not repeat doses if serum osmolality greater than 325 or sodium greater than 155
      - Replace potassium and magnesium lost through diuresis
  - Hypertonic saline
    - Formulations
      - 3% saline
        - 250 to 300 mL bolus over 10 to 20 minutes
        - Administer via central vein ideally, but peripheral is possible
      - 23.4% saline
        - 30 to 60 mL bolus over 10 to 20 minutes
        - Must be administered by central vein
    - Monitor serum sodium
      - Avoid raising by more than 12 mEq/L in 24 h or beyond 160 mEq/L
- Hyperventilation
  - Best performed by increasing the respiratory rate
  - Goal $PaCO_2$ is 30 mm Hg
  - Onset of effect is extremely rapid (minutes)
  - Only useful as a very temporary measure until more definitive therapy is implemented (usually surgical decompression) in severe herniation syndromes
    - Duration of effect is only 30 to 120 minutes
    - Can worsen ischemic brain injury by causing cerebral vasoconstriction when prolonged
  - Should be weaned over hours, in increments of 1 to 2 breaths/minute, to avoid rebound intracranial hypertension

---

on the third day after symptom onset, but it can occur within the first 24 hours.[28,42,45] No historical or neurologic examination findings reliably identify those patients who present without signs of brainstem compression who are at highest risk for deterioration. Imaging findings, however, can be helpful. Not surprisingly, larger infarctions are associated with higher risk. Imaging markers of increased risk of clinical deterioration are listed in **Box 5**.[41,42] Clinical signs of brainstem compression or hydrocephalus are listed in **Table 3**.[28,42] Patients with any of these clinical and imaging markers of

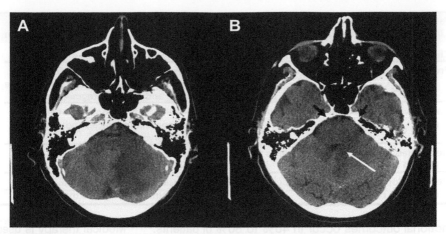

Fig. 3. CT images of a massive cerebellar infarction (*A* and *B*). There is hypodensity in most of the territory of the posterior inferior cerebellar artery (*A* and *B*) with shift of the fourth ventricle away from the side of the infarction (*B, white arrow*) and effacement of the pre-pontine cistern (*B, black arrows*).

elevated risk for deterioration should be admitted to an ICU for continuous neurologic observation.

Examination findings caused by hydrocephalus and those due to brainstem compression overlap substantially, making it very difficult to determine if one or the other is the primary cause of decline. Once any sign of deterioration manifests, the likelihood and rate of progression to severe brainstem compression with coma, cardiorespiratory instability and loss of brainstem reflexes are unpredictable. Progression from the first signs of brainstem compression to coma tends to occur rapidly, over the course of as little as 1 hour and almost always within 24 hours.[28,42] Accordingly, once any risk factor for deterioration due to edema has been identified—and ideally before the first clinical sign of deterioration occurs—neurosurgical consultation must be obtained immediately with the expectation that the patient may need emergent decompression within hours.

Decompressive surgery—external ventricular drainage (EVD) through lateral ventriculostomy and/or suboccipital decompressive craniectomy (SDC)—is life-saving and is the most effective treatment for malignant edema due to a cerebellar infarction. Without surgery, approximately 80% of patients who show signs of brainstem compression die in the short term.[46] In contrast, mortality for patients in coma at the time of surgery who undergo SDC is about 20%,[28,47,48] and good short-term

---

Box 5
Imaging markers of increased risk of clinical deterioration due to massive cerebellar infarction

- Complete territorial infarction or infarction of the median vermian branches of the posterior inferior cerebellar artery (PICA) or the superior cerebellar artery (SCA)

- Hydrocephalus

- Shift of the fourth ventricle away from the side of infarction

- Deformity or anterior displacement of the brainstem

- Effacement of the basal cisterns

difficult to apply to individual patients, however, due to substantial heterogeneity in the anticoagulants and timing of administration across the different trials as well as heterogeneity in stroke etiology within individual trials. The last issue is crucial, as a priori pathophysiologic considerations and lower quality clinical data suggest that anticoagulation in AIS due to some etiologies—especially those associated with a high likelihood of ultraearly recurrence or progression—may be associated with a favorable risk–benefit ratio.[58] For this reason, in consultation with an experienced vascular or critical care neurologist, the emergency physician could consider acute anticoagulation in patients who are not treated with intravenous thrombolysis or endovascular revascularization with AIS due to the mechanisms listed in **Box 7**.[58–66]

Larger infarcts, a higher degree of anticoagulation, and higher blood pressure probably confer a higher risk of the most dreaded complication, ICH.[67,68] These issues must be balanced against the estimated benefit in terms of preventing early recurrent stroke when considering acute anticoagulation in individual patients. For those rare AIS patients for whom anticoagulation is initiated in the ED, exquisite care must be taken to control modifiable factors known to influence the risk of ICH (**Box 8**).

POSTSTROKE SEIZURES

Approximately 5% of AIS patients have a seizure within 7 to 14 days of stroke onset.[69] Most of these seizures are partial, and status epilepticus is particularly uncommon, occurring in less than 1% of patients with AIS. Cortical infarction and higher stroke severity are the only known risk factors for seizures after AIS. It is not clear if the occurrence of early poststroke seizures affects outcome, and the effect of antiseizure prophylaxis has not been well-studied in AIS.[69] On the other hand, some data indicate that exposure to common antiepileptic medications, including phenytoin and benzodiazepines, after AIS seems to worsen long-term neurologic outcome.[70,71] Routine seizure prophylaxis is therefore not recommended after AIS, even in patients with large cortical infarctions. The authors typically treat patients after a first early poststroke seizure with levetiracetam due to its ease of administration, infrequent drug–drug and metabolic interactions, and possible action as a neuroprotective agent.[72] Because of its association with poor neurologic outcomes after stroke, the authors reserve phenytoin for those rare patients with poststroke status epilepticus. The authors' treatment of status epilepticus in AIS patients does not differ from the way they treat this disorder in other patient groups.

SEDATION AND ANALGESIA

Because of the primacy of the neurologic examination in monitoring the physiology of the brain, every reasonable effort must be made to avoid confounding it with sedatives and analgesics. For many AIS patients, this is not an issue as, in the absence of

---

Box 7
Possible indications for acute anticoagulation in AIS

- Symptomatic stenosis or acute occlusion of cervical or large intracranial arteries (internal carotid, vertebral, middle cerebral, and basilar arteries)
- Dissection of a cervical vertebral or internal carotid artery
- Cardoembolism due to mechanical heart valve or intracardiac thrombus (noninfectious etiologies)

Box 8
Method of acute anticoagulation in AIS

- Continuous intravenous infusion of unfractionated heparin. Avoid longer-acting, less easily reversible agents such as warfarin and low molecular weight heparin (LMWH)
- Avoid bolus doses to avoid unpredictable rises in aPTT
- Goal aPTT: 1.5–2 × normal
- Monitor aPTT every 6 hours regardless of stability of previous values
- Maintain blood pressure <180/95 mm Hg
- In the case of neurologic decline: (1) stop heparin infusion, (2) obtain noncontrast head CT, (3) reverse heparin with protamine sulfate in patients with ICH and significant neurologic decline and/or mass effect

---

endotracheal intubation, significant pain and agitation are uncommon problems. Careful thought should be given to the indications for and manner by which sedation and analgesia are achieved in the intubated AIS patient. Many AIS patients, for example, are intubated at least in part due to decreased level of arousal. These patients frequently do not show signs of pain or agitation and should not receive sedatives or analgesics. For those patients who do have significant pain or agitation, non-pharmacologic measures such as optimizing ventilation, treating urinary obstruction, minimizing stimulation, offering reassurance, and when possible, allowing the presence of a person familiar to the patient, should be attempted first.[36]

If these are unsuccessful, the patient should be assessed for pain and, if present, treated with analgesics. The minimal necessary dose of short-acting agents that have the least effect on the neurologic examination should be used. Extreme care should be taken to avoid or counteract the potentially significant hypotensive effects possessed by most of the commonly used sedatives and analgesics. The authors find a step-wise approach that begins with nonsedating agents such as acetaminophen and tramadol to be useful. Revised goals are often necessary for treatment of severe pain in patients with acute brain injuries, as treatment to zero pain without significant alteration of the neurologic examination caused by the analgesics is rarely possible.

If these methods fail to calm an agitated patient, the authors use sedatives following the same basic principles as treatment of pain: start low and go slow. For nonintubated patients, very low doses of antipsychotics or short-acting benzodiazepines are useful. Antipsychotics are the authors' drug of choice owing to their lesser propensity for causing significant sedation, respiratory compromise, and delirium than benzodiazepines. The authors find low-dose quetiapine (12.5 to 25 mg) to be particularly useful. This drug is less likely than haloperidol to cause corrected QT interval prolongation and extrapyramidal symptoms, and has been shown to be quite useful for treating ICU delirium in small studies of non-neurologic patients.[73,74] For patients who do not have enteral access, haloperidol starting at 0.5 to 1.5 mg IM or intravenous every 15 to 30 minutes, with slow dose escalation if the preceding dose was ineffective, can be used. If the agitation appears to be caused predominantly by anxiety, the authors may administer 0.5 to 1 mg of lorazepam intravenously. If this is ineffective after 15 minutes, they will occasionally repeat the dose once more. The authors generally do not give more benzodiazepines than this because of their propensity to significantly confound the neurologic examination.

Propofol is probably the most widely used sedative in neurocritical care for intubated patients because of its extremely short duration of action.[75] When propofol is used in the AIS patient, one must anticipate hypotension and not allow the MAP to drop by more than about 10%. Decreasing the rate of propofol infusion, intravenous boluses of normal saline and vasopressors may be required. The authors avoid midazolam when possible because of its prolonged duration of effect when used as a continuous infusion, particularly in patients with renal or hepatic dysfunction.[76] Dexmedetomidine is a central alpha-2 adrenergic receptor agonist that has nearly ideal properties as a sedating agent for AIS patients; it effectively diminishes agitation and anxiety while depressing consciousness far less than propofol or midazolam, does not significantly blunt respiratory drive, has analgesic properties, and does not frequently lead to significant hypotension.[77] In a number of studies, including 2 large, blinded, randomized, controlled trials, when compared with lorazepam and midazolam for sedation in the general ICU patients, dexmedetomidine has been shown to decrease time with delirium, coma, and mechanical ventilation.[77] It has also been shown to be safe and effective in small studies in critically ill neurologic and neurosurgical patients.[78,79] The main adverse effect of dexmedetomidine is bradycardia, which rarely can be severe. Because dexmedetomidine has not been well-studied, specifically in AIS and other acutely brain-injured patients and these patients may be prone to autonomic instability, vigilance for bradycardia and a low threshold for discontinuation of the drug if bradycardia occurs seem warranted in this context.[80]

CARDIAC CONSIDERATIONS

Cardiac complications are common and explain up to 20% of the early mortality after ischemic stroke.[81,82] Patients with ischemic stroke are at risk for cardiac complications not only due to shared risk factors, but also due to neurogenic factors. One example of the latter would be a patient with a right middle cerebral artery stroke involving the insular cortex, which is associated with a higher risk of cardiac complications thought to be related to disruption of the autonomic nervous system.

An electrocardiogram (EKG) is recommended in all AIS patients due to the high incidence of concomitant heart disease.[2] While EKG abnormalities occur in up to 90% of stroke patients, potentially life-threatening arrhythmias occur in less than 10% of patients.[83] EKG changes such as ST segment and T wave changes are very common in the setting of a stroke and may be difficult to distinguish from acute myocardial infarction. Approximately 13% of ischemic stroke patients have a concomitant myocardial infarction.[83] Particularly for patients who present within the time window for thrombolytitc or endovascular therapy, obtaining an EKG should not be allowed to prolong the time to head CT.

Cardiac troponin levels may be elevated in 17% of patients with ischemic stroke and are associated with higher risk of in-hospital cardiac complications and death.[84] Troponin release may either be due to autonomic activation after AIS (particularly involving the insular cortex) or be due to comorbid coronary artery disease with myocardial ischemia. The TRELAS (TRoponin ELevation in Acute ischemic Stroke) trial will prospectively determine the frequency and potential etiology of troponin elevation in a large cohort of ischemic stroke patients with the intention of providing recommendations for cardiac evaluation of these patients.[85]

Atrial Fibrillation

Atrial fibrillation, which may be either the cause of or the result of the stroke, is probably the most common arrhythmia associated with AIS. Other arrhythmias such as sinus tachycardia and premature ventricular or atrial complexes may be nearly as common. Atrial fibrillation often suggests underlying disease such as myocardial infarction, thyrotoxicosis, and acute lung disease. Atrial fibrillation is associated with higher mortality after AIS.[86] A retrospective review of the Virtual International Stroke Trials Archive-Acute database containing patients from 30 acute stroke trials revealed that atrial fibrillation was associated with a significantly higher rate of serious cardiac complications including heart failure, ventricular tachycardia or fibrillation, and cardiac mortality.[87] Given the higher rate of potentially preventable cardiac complications, close surveillance of those patients with atrial fibrillation is suggested.

Although there are no clinical trials looking at the value of cardiac monitoring in acute stroke patients, AHA/ASA guidelines state that at least 24 hours of telemetry monitoring are warranted to screen for atrial fibrillation or other serious arrhythmias.[2]

Congestive Heart Failure

In AIS, acute myocardial infarction and heart failure have been found to be associated with increased mortality at 3 months.[88] Factors associated with higher risk of in-hospital myocardial infarction or heart failure include history of angina, myocardial infarction in the 3 months before admission, admission hyperglycemia, and high admission NIHSS score.[88] Awareness of these risk factors for cardiac complications may help with timely management and possibly improve clinical outcome.

Similar to findings in other studies, a prospective cohort of over 500 patients with ischemic stroke found elevated serum brain natriuretic peptide (BNP) levels were associated with cardioembolic stroke, lower ejection fraction, left atrial dilatation, and atrial fibrillation. Among those with cardioembolic stroke, elevated BNP was associated with higher mortality and lower likelihood of good functional outcome at 6 months.[86] BNP testing might be considered for prognostication as well as to help determine aggressiveness of heart failure treatment and intensity of monitoring.

Neurogenic Stunned Myocardium

Neurogenic stunned myocardium is a reversible cause of cardiac dysfunction seen more frequently with subarachnoid hemorrhage, but it can occur with other acute intracranial disorders such as ischemic stroke. It is characterized by globally decreased myocardial wall motion not caused by coronary disease, and it is more likely to occur in women and in those with a more severe neurologic injury. It is thought to be caused by a catecholamine surge, which leads to contraction band necrosis.[89] It has been described as tako-tsubo cardiomyopathy due to its appearance similar to that of an octopus fishing pot. Diffuse - as opposed to focal - EKG changes, echocardiographically determined wall-motion abnormalities that do not correlate with a coronary vascular territory, and cardiac troponin levels that are disproportionately low for the degree of ST-segment changes and wall-motion abnormalities can distinguish this reversible condition from a myocardial infarction.[90]

Summary of Cardiac Considerations

Awareness and early recognition of these potential cardiac complications are imperative to avoid delays in treatment. For arrhythmias, treatment would be similar to their treatment in nonstroke patients. Beta-blockers and calcium channel blockers are generally used to reduce a rapid ventricular rate. Cardiology consultation should be considered. For neurogenic stunned myocardium with significant depression of left ventricular function, avoidance of fluid overload, supportive care including in rare cases inotropic drugs, and treatment of causal neurologic issues such as intracranial hypertension may be helpful. If inotropic support is needed, milrinone offers the theoretical advantage over dobutamine in that it is not an adrenergic receptor agonist, a potentially important consideration given the role of catecholamine excess in the generation of neurogenic stress myocardium.[91]

PULMONARY CONSIDERATIONS
Respiratory Failure

Respiratory failure occurs in about 5% to 10% of AIS patients,[92,93] and up to 25% of patients with infarction in the MCA territory.[94,95] It is most frequently caused by loss of airway control, itself the result of a combination of decreased arousal and orophrayng-eal incoordination. These lead to impaired handling of secretions and inefficient respiratory mechanics due to collapse of the upper airway.[96] Patients with basilar territory infarctions additionally may have central hypoventilation with periods of apnea.[97] Pulmonary parenchymal disease is less common and is typically due to aspiration pneumonitis/pneumonia, and rarely neurogenic pulmonary edema.

Respiratory failure has critical consequences for AIS patients, as both hypercapnea and hypoxemia can worsen brain injury through worsening ischemic injury and raising the ICP. Accordingly, it must be detected and reversed as early as possible. This is made challenging by the fact that the presentation and evolution of respiratory failure in AIS often differ considerably from that seen in patients with acute pulmonary disease.[96] Rather than manifesting obvious signs such as anxiety, tachypnea, increased respiratory effort, and low oxygen saturation, AIS patients in respiratory failure frequently have depressed arousal, a respiratory pattern that may not appear labored, and, as long as supplemental oxygen is supplied, oxygen saturation readings that can remain normal until late. If allowed to continue, through a vicious cycle of hypoventilation, secretion accumulation, atelectasis, hypoxemia, and hypercapnea, this process can insidiously lead to cardiopulmonary collapse with refractory hypoxemia, bradycardia, hypotension, and cardiac arrest.[98]

Determination of the need for endotracheal intubation in AIS, therefore, is based largely on indications other than oxygen saturation and findings on chest imaging and arterial blood gas testing. Thus far, there are no evidence-based guidelines for the optimal timing and specific indications for intubation in AIS, and the decision remains based on clinical judgment. Specific relative indications are listed in **Box 9**.

Once the AIS patient has been determined to have respiratory failure, if a rapidly correctable cause is not present, he or she should undergo endotracheal intubation. Noninvasive positive pressure ventilation should not be used in these patients, as it does not correct the underlying problems with airway control and, in fact, can exacerbate them.[99]

Technique of Rapid Sequence Intubation

The consequences of the physiologic disturbances that commonly occur during rapid sequence intubation are amplified in the AIS patient. Hypoxemia, hypercapnea, hypertension, and hypotension can all exacerbate ischemic brain injury. Additionally,

---

Box 9
Relative indications for tracheal intubation in AIS patients

- Decreased or rapidly progressive decline in level of arousal. A GCS of 8 to 10 has been proposed as a trigger, but the GCS is not an ideal measurement tool in AIS patients.

- Weakness or incoordination of the facial, oral, lingual, and pharyngeal musculature and reflexes. Key signs on examination include prominent facial weakness, severe dysarthria, obstructed respiratory pattern/sounds, weak/absent cough, and poor handling of oral secretions (drooling, pharyngeal pooling)

- Large hemispheric or cerebellar infarctions

- Brainstem infarctions, especially in the pons

airway manipulation and succinylcholine have the potential to transiently lead to significant elevation of the ICP,[100,101] a crucial concern for patients with space-occupying infarcts.

Intubation techniques generally do not differ for AIS patients and are beyond the scope of this article. However, a few issues surrounding the choice of drugs in RSI for AIS are worth noting (**Table 4**).[100–104]

Strategies for Mechanical Ventilation

Mechanical ventilation of AIS patients is generally simple due to their typical lack of coexisting acute pulmonary disease.[96] Oxygenation is paramount. Although there is no clear evidence to support any specific oxygenation targets, the authors aim to keep the oxygen saturation greater than 94% and the PaO2 greater than 80 mm Hg to facilitate oxygen delivery to ischemic brain. Hyperoxygenation with normobaric

Table 4
Issues regarding rapid sequence intubation technique in AIS

Phase of Rapid Sequence Intubation	Issues
Premedication	Airway manipulation can potently elevate ICP. Premedication with lidocaine (1.5 mg/kg intravenously) and fentanyl (2.5–3.0 µg/kg intravenously) can significantly blunt this response and should be performed when possible. Higher dose fentanyl boluses, which have been associated with transient but substantial increases in ICP and decreases in cerebral perfusion pressure, should not be used
Induction	Etomidate is the ideal induction agent for most AIS patients owing to its minimal hemodynamic effects while remaining effective at creating favorable intubating conditions. Ketamine, which generally raises the blood pressure by way of sympathetic stimulation, is an alternative that can be considered in hypotensive patients. Older evidence indicating that ketamine causes an elevation in ICP has been contradicted by newer studies, although none have examined ketamine's effect on ICP specifically during RSI
Paralysis	Succinylcholine has been associated with elevations in ICP. While this issue is controversial, it deserves consideration in patients with large, space-occupying infarctions, for whom this effect could at least theoretically lead to significant intracranial hypertension, cerebral hypoperfusion, and even herniation. Additionally, AIS patients not infrequently present to the ED after having been down in the field for prolonged times, placing them at risk for rhabdomyolysis, an important contraindication to the use of succinylcholine. In either of these 2 scenarios, consideration should be given to either using a defasciculating dose of a nondepolarizing agent before paralysis with succinylcholine or to using a rapid-onset nondepolarizing agent such as rocuronium

and hyperbaric techniques are currently being investigated as therapies for AIS. Because thus far there is no high-quality supportive clinical evidence, these techniques should not be used outside of research protocols.[105]

Even in patients with considerable cerebral edema, prophylactic hyperventilation is not useful and potentially harmful due to, respectively, its short-lived effect on intracranial pressure and potential to exacerbate cerebral ischemia. Hypercapnea, a potent cause of increased ICP, must be fastidiously avoided. The authors' PaCO2 goal in mechanically ventilated patients, therefore, is in the low normal range of 37 to 42 mm Hg.

RENAL CONSIDERATIONS
Intravascular Volume Targets

The importance of adequate intravascular volume in AIS has already been discussed. The goal for fluid management is euvolemia, as hypervolemia has enough negative consequences for the pulmonary and nervous systems to make it nearly as undesirable as hypovolemia. As in other critically ill patients, determination of intravascular euvolemia can be difficult in AIS patients. Blood pressure in the target range for the patient, heart rate less than 100 beats per minute, normal serum urea nitrogen (BUN) and creatinine, a BUN–creatinine ratio less than 20, and urine output at least 0.5 mL/kg/h are all markers of euvolemia. Consistent with studies in other types of critically ill patients, the authors do not find that measurement of central venous pressure or hemodynamic indices obtained from a pulmonary artery catheter is useful in managing the volume status and hemodynamics of AIS patients who do not have concomitant major derangements of cardiovascular system function.[106,107]

Choice of Intravenous Fluid Solution

Normal saline is essentially the only intravenous fluid solution that should be used for intravascular volume augmentation and maintenance in AIS patients. More hypotonic formulations, such as 0.45% saline and Lactated Ringer solution, are almost never used, because they do not augment or maintain intravascular volume as well as normal saline and, by virtue of their lower osmolality, can worsen cerebral edema.[108,109] While intermittent bolus administration of hypertonic saline solutions such as 3% saline can be useful for treating intracranial hypertension, their value as a continuous infusion is unclear.[110,111] The authors reserve continuous infusions of hypertonic saline for the treatment of severe hyponatremia. Dextrose-containing solutions of any osmolality should be reserved for the treatment of hypoglycemia because of the well-established and diverse deleterious effects of elevated serum glucose on acute cerebral infarctions. There is at present no role for routine administration of intravenous colloid solutions. Although the effectiveness of albumin infusion early in AIS as a neuroprotective therapy is currently being investigated, lack of high-quality human clinical data indicating benefit and possible problems with safety preclude the use of albumin infusions in the routine care of AIS patients.[112]

Electrolyte Management

Magnesium has been shown to have neuroprotective effects in a number of animal models. Clear clinical evidence of the effectiveness of magnesium supplementation in improving outcomes after AIS is thus far lacking. Safety of moderate magnesium supplementation, on the other hand, appears to be acceptable.[113] Accordingly, it is the authors' practice to maintain high-normal magnesium concentrations of 2 to 2.5 mg/dL in AIS patients through the use of intravenous magnesium sulfate infusions.

The effect, if any, of serum potassium concentration on AIS outcomes has not been well investigated. Extrapolating from epidemiologic data linking low serum potassium concentration with increased risk of stroke mortality as well as recent data linking increased mortality in acute myocardial infarction with serum potassium concentrations less than 3.5 mEq/L or greater than 4.5 mEq/L, the authors aim to maintain a serum potassium concentration of 3.5 to 4.5 mEq/L in their AIS patients.[114,115] Because of changes in osmolality associated with changes in serum sodium concentration, serum sodium levels should be maintained within normal limits. Sodium concentration abnormalities are common in AIS, but a detailed discussion of their diagnosis and management is beyond the scope of this article. Interested readers are referred to the review by Rabinstein and Wijdicks.[116]

TEMPERATURE CONTROL

Induced hypothermia has been recognized as being potentially beneficial in limiting secondary injury after acute brain injury since the middle of the 20th century.[117] More recently, human and animal data have consistently shown that even low levels of fever can significantly worsen ischemic brain injury.[118] In the Copenhagen Stroke Study, a large prospective cohort study of predominantly AIS patients, a 1°C increase in body temperature on admission doubled the odds of in-hospital death or poor neurologic outcome at discharge, independent of other, known predictors of outcome.[119] These observations are explained by the fact that most of the key cellular and molecular processes underlying secondary brain injury—including apoptosis, mitochondrial dysfunction, endothelial dysfunction, inflammation, and excitotoxicity—are temperature-dependent.[117] These facts, along with the success of therapeutic hypothermia in improving outcomes after cardiac arrest and perinatal asphyxia,[117] have intensified investigation of induced normothermia (IN) and therapeutic hypothermia (TH) as treatments for AIS.

Induced Normothermia

IN is the use of pharmacologic fever control and physical cooling therapies to maintain normothermia (37 to 37.5°C) in patients with fever. Small, preliminary human clinical studies of IN in patients with severe brain injury of various types have shown the therapy to reduce intracranial pressure and microdialysis markers of cerebral metabolic distress.[120,121] Nonetheless, there are at present no clinical data directly relating the effect of IN on neurologic outcome in patients with brain injury of any type, including AIS. Accordingly, the indirect evidence provided by studies identifying fever as a strong risk factor for poor neurologic outcome along with the relative ease and safety of application of IN with recently developed surface and endovascular cooling devices underlie the rationale for using IN in AIS patients.[118]

IN is associated with adverse effects that are similar to those seen with TH, perhaps the most important of which is shivering. Shivering, caused by activation of the sympathetic nervous system, not only limits the effectiveness of fever control therapies in lowering body temperature, but also increases the total body metabolic rate by as much as a factor of 3; additionally, it is associated with a rise in mean arterial pressure of about 10 mm Hg. Although these responses are most common and potent in young, male patients, they are of the most consequence in older patients of either sex, in whom the hemodynamic consequences of these physiologic changes can have serious cardiovascular consequences.[122] In addition, shivering may increase the cerebral metabolic rate, and in patients with severe brain injury, shivering is associated with increased intracranial pressure and decreased brain tissue oxygenation.[123] For all of these reasons, effective shiver control is paramount to effectively employing

IN. The masking of fever as an indication of new or worsening infection and the possibility of worsening of existing infections are other important adverse effects of IN.

The authors employ IN in patients with large ischemic strokes for neuroprotection and to limit cerebral edema using a step-wise approach. The first step, which can be easily employed in the ED, involves simple environmental interventions (minimal clothing/bed clothes on the patient and a cool room) and administration of acetaminophen. The authors do not use a typical cooling blanket as, in their experience, these often produce shivering without significantly lowering the core temperature. The next step is active temperature control using the Arctic Sun external cooling device (Medivance, Louisville, Colorado). At this point. an antishivering protocol based on the Columbia ant-shivering protocol is used.[124] Given the lack of clear benefit of IN, the authors abort the treatment if shivering cannot be controlled without the use of neuromuscular blocking agents unless it appears to be controlling potentially malignant cerebral edema. Given its complexity, labor-intensive nature, potentially narrow therapeutic index with shivering, and unknown benefits, the authors do not take IN beyond environmental measures and acetaminophen in the ED.

Therapeutic Hypothermia

There are 2 potential uses for TH in AIS: general neuroprotection and control of malignant cerebral edema.[125] Despite substantial animal evidence for effectiveness in neuroprotection, there are as yet insufficient human clinical data to support the broad use of TH in AIS outside of clinical trials. As of the writing of Polderman's 2008 review, only 145 subjects had been included in 7 small studies of the use of TH in AIS.[117] Since then, the only study of significance published on the topic, the Intravenous Thrombolysis Plus Hypothermia for Acute Treatment of Ischemic Stroke trial, included 59 patients.[126] These existing studies indicate that implementation of TH for AIS patients is feasible, not prohibitively unsafe, and can be combined with intravenous thrombolysis without major hemorrhagic complications.[126–128] Major problems limiting the conclusions that can be drawn from these studies include insufficient numbers of patients for determining effects on clinical outcomes; an excess of potentially preventable adverse effects in treated patients, including infections (mostly pneumonia) and rebound intracranial hypertension during rewarming; differences in duration of hypothermia; and a wide variety of methods and protocols used to control body temperature and shivering and protect against known complications of the therapy. Furthermore, in many studies hypothermia may have been achieved too late to be effective. Based on animal data, this window may be as short as 1 hour, and at its longest probably is not longer than 6 hours.[117] Given the widespread experience and success achieved with the use of TH for coma after cardiac arrest and the lessons learned in these preliminary studies, the time is ripe for a large-scale trial of TH for AIS.

While the utility of routine use of TH in AIS is unknown, existing data rather clearly show that malignant cerebral edema and elevated ICP can be effectively controlled by TH.[117,127] Accordingly, TH may be useful in treating AIS patients with malignant edema who either cannot undergo hemicraniectomy or for whom hemicraniectomy fails to control intracranial hypertension or shift. Rebound intracranial hypertension during rewarming is particularly common and dangerous in such patients.[127] Very slow, controlled rewarming at a rate of 0.1°C per hour may prevent this.[129]

GLYCEMIC CONTROL

Hyperglycemia is common in patients arriving to the ED with stroke. Serum glucose greater than 200 mg/dL is associated with a worsened prognosis and has been associated with increased risk of hemorrhagic transformation after thrombolysis.[130,131] Hyperglycemia may be harmful due to increased tissue acidosis, free radical production, impairment of the blood–brain barrier, augmentation of cerebral edema, and higher risk of hemorrhagic transformation of the stroke.[130,132] Another consideration, however, is that hyperglycemia may simply be an epiphenomenon or marker of a more severe stroke.[133]

Persistent hyperglycemia greater than 200 mg/dL during the first 24 hours after a stroke has been shown to predict expansion of the infarct size and poor neurologic outcome.[134] This implies that acute management of hyperglycemia might benefit the AIS patient. The exact blood glucose level that should be targeted, however, is not entirely clear. In the AHA/ASA ischemic stroke guideline, a class 2a, level C evidence recommendation is to administer insulin when serum glucose concentration is greater than 140 to 185 mg/dL.[2] However, since that guideline was published, the NICE-SUGAR (Normoglycemia in Intensive Care Evaluation-Survival Using Glucose Algorithm) trial of critically ill medical and surgical patients found higher mortality with target blood glucose levels of 80 to 110 mg/dL compared with levels of 140 to 180 mg/dL.[135] This trial did not, however, report inclusion of ischemic stroke patients. One small prospective randomized trial of insulin for glycemic control in critically ill neurologic patients (including ischemic stroke patients) found no difference in neurologic outcome when a goal of serum glucose less than 151 mg/dL was compared with a goal of 80 to 110 mg/dL. There was a higher incidence of hypoglycemia in the group with the lower goal glucose concentration.[136] It is hoped that further evidence from ongoing trials, such as the Stroke Hyperglycemia Insulin Network Effort (SHINE) trial will clarify the risk–benefit analysis of glycemic control in AIS.

Because hypoglycemia can mimic AIS signs and can lead to irreversible brain injury, close monitoring for this complication and rapid treatment when it is detected are essential. Concerns have been raised in microdialysis studies that intensive glycemic control may lead to low cerebral extracellular glucose and be detrimental to severely brain injured patients.[137] Given the dual concerns of potential hypoglycemia and its consequences with intensive insulin therapy on the 1 hand, and the importance of avoiding severe hyperglycemia on the other, the authors' approach is to administer insulin aiming for a blood glucose level of 120 to 180 mg/dL with close glucose monitoring. A continuous infusion of intravenous insulin is preferred in critically ill patients, while subcutaneous insulin may be appropriate in most other patients.

PROPHYLAXIS
Pneumonia

Pneumonia develops in about 13% of AIS patients, and causes approximately 35% of deaths after AIS.[138] Fortunately, this is largely a preventable complication. Dysphagia, which may occur in up to 78% of stroke patients, is thought to be responsible for a large proportion of poststroke pneumonia by way of aspiration of oral and gastric contents.[138,139] Despite well-established risk factors, poststroke aspiration is infrequently clinically obvious, and many patients without overt oropharyngeal dysfunction are at risk for clinically significant dysphagia and aspiration.[138,139] Hinchey and colleagues demonstrated that use of a formal dysphagia screen, leading to withholding or modification of oral intake for patients with dysphagia, was associated with a >50% reduction in poststroke pneumonia.[138] As stroke-related dysphagia tends to be worst early in the illness, it is crucial for its detection to occur as early in a patient's hospital course as possible. This makes the ED the ideal place for dysphagia screening. Dysphagia screening is simple, consisting of observing a patient swallow a small amount of water.[140] It can be performed at the bedside by any nurse or physician trained in the evaluation. Current AHA/ASA guidelines recommend that no oral intake, including medications such as aspirin, be allowed in AIS unless the patient passes a bedside dysphagia screen. Adherence to this recommendation is an important quality indicator for AIS stroke care. For patients who fail the bedside dysphagia screen, consideration should be given to placing a nasogastric tube in the ED (contraindicated if the patient has received rt-PA) if oral medications are necessary.

Venous Thromboembolism

In the absence of venous thromboembolism (VTE) prophylaxis, approximately 25% to 68% of AIS patients will develop a deep venous thrombosis (DVT) or pulmonary embolus (PE).[141] This risk increases up to 75% in patients with hemiplegia.[142] DVTs may develop as early as poststroke day 2, with peak incidence occurring between poststroke days 2 and 7. Pulmonary emboli account for about 20% of VTE complications in AIS and are estimated to cause 25% of early deaths following AIS.[142] Accordingly, careful, early VTE prophylaxis is crucial. The use of subcutaneous unfractionated heparin (UFH) or LMWH has been associated with a 79% decrease in risk of DVT and a 40% decrease in risk of symptomatic PE.[142] The effectiveness of intermittent sequential compression devices (SCDs) in AIS is unclear, but they have few adverse effects.[143] VTE prophylaxis should consist of immediate application of SCDs to the lower limbs and early (generally beginning 12 to 24 hours after admission) mobilization with at least passive range of motion exercises. Prophylactic subcutaneous UFH or LWMH should begin immediately for all patients except those with strong contraindications. Patients who received intravenous rt-PA should receive a first dose of prophylactic UFH or LMWH 24 hours after the rt-PA was administered, provided there is no major hemorrhagic transformation on follow-up CT.[2]

Stress Ulcer

Critically ill AIS patients are under the influence of similar physiologic stressors as other critically ill patients. They may actually have increased gastric mucosal destruction associated with increased vagal tone and greater gastric acid production.[144] While there is a relative paucity of data related specifically to the risk of stress ulcers and effectiveness of prophylaxis in stroke patients, it is reasonable to extrapolate from the general ICU and traumatic brain injury data and conclude that critically ill AIS patients are at high enough risk to warrant active prophylaxis. Such prophylaxis should consist of the use of either a proton pump inhibitor or histamine type-2 receptor antagonist and early (within 24 hours of admission) enteral feeding.[144]

PROGNOSIS

Early prognostication in the setting of AIS lacks precision and accuracy. The consequences of early rendering of a dismal prognosis, however, can be absolute, influencing decisions about level and aggression of care for the patient's family as well as for other members of the medical team.[145] Even in the setting of more severe ischemic stroke syndromes, including the malignant MCA syndrome or basilar artery occlusion, poor outcomes are not guaranteed. Early establishment of a poor prognosis in the ED might lead to premature limitations in treatment or early withdrawal of care, resulting in a self-fulfilling prophecy of poor outcome.[146] Although one can never be sure that if such patients were offered more aggressive treatment their outcomes would be better, enough uncertainty surrounds early prognostication that it is generally not advisable to make definitive neurologic prognoses in the emergency room setting regarding AIS patients.

REFERENCES

1. Saver JL. Time is brain—quantified. Stroke 2006;37:263–6.
2. Adams HP Jr, del Zoppo G, Alberts MJ, et al. Guidelines for the early management of adults with ischemic stroke. Stroke 2007;38:1655–711.
3. Reeves MJ, Arora S, Broderick JP. Acute stroke care in the US: results from 4 pilot prototypes of the Paul Coverdell national acute stroke registry. Stroke 2005;36:1232–40.
4. Rincon F, Mayer SA, Rivolta J. Impact of delayed transfer of critically ill stroke patients from the emergency department to the neuro-ICU. Neurocrit Care 2010;13:75–81.
5. Nguyen T, Koroshetz WJ. Intensive care management of ischemic stroke. Curr Neurol Neurosci Rep 2003;3:32–9.
6. Wartenberg KE, Schmidt M, Mayer SA. Multimodality monitoring in neurocritical care. Crit Care Clin 2007;23:507–38.
7. Hillered L, Vespa PM, Hovda DA. Translational neurochemical research in acute human brain injury: the current status and potential future for cerebral microdialysis. J Neurotrauma 2005;22:3–41.
8. Kasner SE. Clinical interpretation and use of stroke scales. Lancet Neurol 2006; 5:603–12.
9. Wijdicks EF, Bamlet WR, Maramattom BV, et al. Validation of a new coma scale: the FOUR score. Ann Neurol 2005;58:585–93.
10. Idrovo L, Fuentes B, Medina J, et al. Validation of the FOUR score (Spanish version) in acute stroke: an interobserver variability study. Eur Neurol 2010;63: 364–9.
11. Kornbluth J, Bhardwaj A. Evaluation of coma: a critical appraisal of popular scoring systems. Neurocrit Care 2011;14:134–43.
12. Stead LG, Wijdicks EF, Bhagra A, et al. Validation of a new coma scale, the FOUR score, in the emergency department. Neurocrit Care 2009;10:50–4.
13. Rose JC, Mayer SA. Optimizing blood pressure in neurological emergencies. Neurocrit Care 2004;3:287–300.
14. Qureshi AI. Acute hypertensive response in patients with stroke: pathophysiology and management. Circulation 2008;118:176–87.
15. Sandset EC, Bath PM, Boysen G, et al. The angiotensin-receptor blocker candesartan for treatment of acute stroke (SCAST): a randomised, placebo-controlled, double-blind trial. Lancet 2011;377:741–50.
16. Mayer SA, Kurtz P, Wyman A, et al. Clinical practices, complications, and mortality in neurological patients with acute severe hypertension: the studying the treatment of acute hypertension (STAT) registry. Crit Care Med 2011;39:2330–6.
17. Oliveira-Fihlo J, Silva SC, Trabuco CC, et al. Detrimental effects of blood pressure reduction in the first 24 hours of acute stroke onset. Neurology 2003;61: 1047–51.
18. van Mook WN, Rennenberg RJ, Schurink GW, et al. Cerebral hyperperfusion syndrome. Lancet Neurol 2005;4:877–8.
19. Barer DH, Cruickshank JM, Ebrahim SB, et al. Low dose beta blockade in acute stroke ("BEST" trial): an evaluation. BMJ 1988;296:737–41.
20. Mistri AK, Robinson TG, Potter JF. Pressor therapy in acute ischemic stroke: a systematic review. Stroke 2006;37:1565–71.

21. Rodriguez GJ, Cordina SM, Vazquez G, et al. The hydration influence on risk of stroke (THIRST) study. Neurocrit Care 2009;10:187–94.
22. Bhalla A, Sankaralingam S, Dundas R, et al. Influence of raised plasma osmolality on clinical outcome after acute stroke. Stroke 2000;31:2043–8.
23. Aicher FT, Fazekas F, Brainin M, et al. Hypervolemic hemodilution in acute ischemic stroke: the multicenter Austrian hemodilution stroke trial (MAHST). Stroke 1998;29:743–9.
24. Wojner-Alexander AW, Garani Z, Chenyshev OY, et al. Heads down: flat positioning improves blood flow velocity in acute ischemic stroke. Neurology 2005;64:1354–7.
25. Schwarz S, Georgiadis D, Aschoff A, et al. Effects of body position on intracranial pressure and cerebral perfusion in patients with large hemispheric stroke. Stroke 2002;33:497–501.
26. Drakulovic MB, Torres A, Bauer TT, et al. Supine body position as a risk factor for nosocomial pneumonia in mechanically ventilated patients: a randomised trial. Lancet 1999;354:1851–8.
27. Wijdicks EF. "Comatose". The practice of emergency and critical care neurology. Oxford (United Kingdom): Oxford University Press; 2010.
28. Hornig CR, Rust DS, Busse O, et al. Space-occupying cerebellar infarction. Clinical course and prognosis. Strok 1994;25:372–4.
29. Hacke W, Schwab S, Horn M. "Malignant" middle cerebral artery territory infarction: clinical course and prognostic signs. Arch Neurol 1996;53:309–15.
30. Manno EM, Nichols DR, Fulgham JR, et al. Computed tomographic determinants of neurologic deterioration in patients with large middle cerebral artery infarctions. Mayo Clin Proc 2003;78:156–60.
31. Frank JI. Large hemispheric infarction, deterioration, and intracranial pressure. Neurology 1995;45:1286–90.
32. Huttner HB, Schwab S. Malignant middle cerebral artery infarction: clinical characteristics, treatment strategies, and future perspectives. Lancet Neurol 2009;8:949–58.
33. Moulin T, Cattin F, Crepin-Leblond T, et al. Early CT signs in acute middle cerebral artery infarction: predictive value for subsequent infarct locations and outcome. Neurology 1996;47:366–75.
34. Wijdicks EF, Diringer MN. Middle cerebral artery territory infarction and early brain swelling: progression and effect of age on outcome. Mayo Clin Proc 1998;73:829–36.
35. Hofmeijer J, Kappelle LJ, Algra A, et al. Surgical decompression for space-occupying cerebral infarction (the hemicraniectomy after middle cerebral artery infarction with life-threatening edema trial [HAMLET]): a multicentre, open, randomised trial. Lancet Neurol 2009;8:326–33.
36. Wijdicks EF. Intracranial pressure. The practice of emergency and critical care neurology. Oxford (United Kingdom): Oxford University Press; 2010.
37. Koenig MA, Bryan M, Lewin JL, et al. Reversal of transtentorial herniation with hypertonic saline. Neurology 2008;70:1023–9.
38. Kamal H, Navi BB, Nakagawa K, et al. Hypertonic saline versus mannitol for the treatment of elevated intracranial pressure: a meta-analysis of randomized clinical trials. Crit Care Med 2011;39:554–9.
39. Juttler E, Schwab S, Schmiedek P, et al. Decompressive surgery for the treatment of malignant infarction of the middle cerebral artery (DESTINY): a randomized, controlled trial. Stroke 2007;38:2518–25.

40. Vahedi K, Vicaut E, Mateo J, et al. Sequential-design, multicenter, randomized, controlled trial of early decompressive craniectomy in malignant middle cerebral artery infarction (DECIMAL Trial). Stroke 2007;38:2506–17.
41. Koh MG, Phan TG, Atkinson JL, et al. Neuroimaging in deteriorating patients with cerebellar infarcts and mass effect. Stroke 2000;31:2062–7.
42. Kase CS, Norrving B, Levine SR, et al. Cerebellar infarction. Clinical and anatomic observation in 66 cases. Stroke 1993;24:76–83.
43. Amarenco P. The spectrum of cerebellar infarctions. Neurology 1991;41:973–9.
44. Macdonnell RA, Kalnins RN, Donnan GA. Cerebellar infarction: natural history, prognosis, and pathology. Stroke 1987;18:849–55.
45. Jauss M, Krieger D, Hornig C, et al. Surgical and medical management of patients with massive cerebellar infarctions: results of the German-Austrian cerebellar infarction study. J Neurol 1997;246:257–64.
46. Heros RC. Cerebellar hemorrhage and infarction. Stroke 1982;13:106–9.
47. Juttler E, Schweikert S, Ringleb PA, et al. Long-term outcome after surgical treatment for space-occupying cerebellar infarction: experience in 56 patients. Stroke 2009;40:3060–6.
48. Pfefferkorn T, Eppinger U, Linn J, et al. Long-term outcome after suboccipital decompressive craniectomy for malignant cerebellar infarction. Stroke 2009; 40:3045–50.
49. Wijdicks EF. Cerebellar infarct. The practice of emergency and critical care neurology. Oxford (United Kingdom): Oxford University Press; 2010.
50. The National Institute for Neurological Disorders and Stroke rt-PA Stroke Study Group. Tissue plasminogen activator for acute ischemic stroke. N Engl J Med 1995;333:1581–7.
51. Sussman BJ, Fitch TS. Thrombolysis with fibrinolysin in cerebral arterial occlusion. JAMA 1958;167:1705–9.
52. Meyer JS, Gilroy J, Barnhart MI, et al. Therapeutic thrombolysis in cerebral thromboembolism: double-blind evaluation of intravenous plasmin therapy in carotid and middle cerebral arterial occlusion. Neurology 1963;13:927–37.
53. Katzan IL, Furlan AJ, Lloyd LE, et al. Use of tissue-type plasminogen activator for acute ischemic stroke: the Cleveland area experience. JAMA 2000;283: 1151–8.
54. Engleter ST, Fluri F, Buitrago-Tellez C, et al. Life-threatening orolingual angioedema during thrombolysis in acute ischemic stroke. J Neurol 2005;252:1167–70.
55. Hill MD, Lye T, Moss H, et al. Hemi-orolingual angioedema and ACE inhibition after alteplase treatment of stroke. Neurology 2003;60:1525–7.
56. Hill MD, Barber PA, Takahashi J. Anaphylactoid reactions and angioedema during alteplase treatment of acute ischemic stroke. CMAJ 2000;162:1281–4.
57. Sandercock PA, Counsell C, Kamal AK. Anticoagulants for acute ischemic stroke. Cochrane Database Syst Rev 2008;(8):CD000024.
58. Albers GW, Amaerenco P, Easton JD, et al. Antithrombotic and thrombolytic therapy for ischemic stroke: American College of Chest Physicians evidence-based clinical practice guidelines (8th edition). Chest 2008;133: 630S–69S.
59. Schonewille WJ, Algra A, Serena J, et al. Outcome in patients treated with basilar artery occlusion conventionally. J Neurol Neurosurg Psychiatry 2005; 76:1238–41.
60. Schonewille WJ, Wijman CA, Michel P, et al. Treatment and outcomes in acute basilar artery occlusion in the basilar artery international cooperation study (BASICS): a prospective registry study. Lancet Neurol 2009;8:724–30.

103. Zed PJ, Abu-Laban RB, Harrison DW. Intubating conditions and hemodynamic effects of etomidate for rapid sequence intubation in the emergency department: an observational cohort study. Acad Emerg Med 2006;13:378–83.

104. Filanovsky Y, Miller P, Kao J. Myth: ketamine should not be used as an induction agent for intubation in patients with head injury. CJEM 2010;12:154–7.

105. Michalski D, Hartig W, Schneider D, et al. Use of normobaric and hyperbaric oxygen in acute focal cerebral ischemia—a preclinical and clinical review. Acta Neurol Scand 2011;123:85–97.

106. Marik PE, Baram M, Vahid B. Does central venous pressure predict fluid responsiveness: a systematic review of the literature and the tale of seven mares. Chest 2008;134:172–8.

107. Haidan M, Pinsky MR. Evidence-based review of the use of the pulmonary artery catheter: impact data and complications. Crit Care 2006;10(Suppl 3):S8.

108. Simma B, Burger R, Falk M. A prospective, randomized, and controlled study of fluid management in children with severe head injury: lactated ringer's solution versus hypertonic saline. Crit Care Med 1998;26:1265–70.

109. Ramming S, Schackford SR, Zhuang J, et al. The relationship of fluid balance and sodium administration to cerebral edema formation and intracranial pressure in a porcine model of brain injury. J Trauma 1994;37:705–13.

110. Ziai WC, Tuong TJ, Bhardwaj A. Hypertonic saline: first-line therapy for cerebral edema? J Neurol Sci 2007;261:157–66.

111. Bhardwaj A, Harkuni I, Murphy SJ, et al. Hypertonic saline worsens infarct volume after transient cerebral ischemia in rats. Stroke 2000;31:1694–701.

112. Ginsberg MD, Palesch YY, Martin RH, et al. The albumin in acute stroke (ALIAS) multicenter clinical trial: safety analysis of part 1 and rationale and design of part 2. Stroke 2011;42:119–27.

113. Sahota P, Savitz SI. Investigational therapies for ischemic stroke: neuroprotection and neurorecovery. Neurotherapeutics 2011;8:434–51.

114. Goyal A, Spertus JA, Gosch K, et al. Serum potassium levels and mortality in acute myocardial infarction. JAMA 2012;307:157–64.

115. Green DM, Ropper AH, Kronmal RA, et al. Serum potassium level and dietary potassium intake as risk factors for stroke. Neurology 2002;59:314–20.

116. Rabinstein AA, Wijdicks EF. Hyponatremia in critically ill neurologic patients. Neurologist 2003;9:290–300.

117. Polderman KH. Induced hypothermia and fever control for prevention and treatment of neurological injuries. Lancet 2008;371:1955–69.

118. Badjatia N. Hyperthermia and fever control in brain injury. Crit Care Med 2009; 37(Suppl 7):S250–7.

119. Reith J, Jorgensen HS, Pedersen PM, et al. Body temperature in acute stroke: relation to stroke severity, infarct size, mortality, and outcome. Lancet 1996; 347:422–5.

120. Puccio AM, Fischer MR, Jankowitz BT, et al. Induced normothermia attenuates intracranial hypertension and reduces fever burden after severe traumatic brain injury. Neurocrit Care 2009;11:82–7.

121. Oddo M, Frangos S, Milby A, et al. Induced normothermia attenuates cerebral metabolic distress in patients with aneurysmal subarachnoid hemorrhage and refractory fever. Stroke 2009;40:1913–6.

122. Sessler DI. Thermoregulatory defense mechanisms. Crit Care Med 2009; 37(Suppl 7):S203–10.

123. Oddo M. Effect of shivering on brain tissue oxygenation during induced normothermia in patients with severe brain injury. Neurocrit Care 2010;12:10–6.

124. Choi HA, Ko SB, Presciutti M, et al. Prevention of shivering during therapeutic temperature modulation: the Columbia anti-shivering protocol. Neurocrit Care 2011;14:389–94.

125. Linares G, Mayer SA. Hypothermia for the treatment of ischemic and hemorrhagic stroke. Crit Care Med 2009;37(Suppl 7):S243–9.

126. Hemmen TM, Raman R, Guluma KZ, et al. Intravenous thrombolysis plus hypothermia for acute treatment of ischemic stroke (ICTuS-L): final results. Stroke 2010;41:2265–70.

127. Schwab S, Georgiadis D, Berrouschot J, et al. Feasibility and safety of moderate hypothermia after massive hemispheric infarction. Stroke 2001;32:2033–5.

128. De Georgia MA, Krieger DW, Abou-Chebl A, et al. Cooling of acute ischemic brain damage (COOL-AID): a feasibility trial of endovascular cooling. Neurology 2004;63:312–7.

129. Steiner T, Freide T, Aschoff A, et al. Effect and feasibility of controlled rewarming after moderate hypothermia in stroke patients with malignant infarction of the middle cerebral artery. Stroke 2001;32:2833–5.

130. Kase CS, Furlan AJ, Wechsler LR, et al. Cerebral hemorrhage after intra-arterial thrombolysis for ischemic stroke: the PROACT II trial. Neurology 2001;57:1603–10.

131. Demchuck AM, Morganstern LB, Krieger DW, et al. Serum glucose level and diabetes predict tissue plasminogen activator-related intracerebral hemorrhage in acute ischemic stroke. Stroke 1999;30:34–9.

132. Lindsberg PJ, Roine RO. Hyperglycemia in acute stroke. Stroke 2004;35:363–4.

133. Candelise L, Landi G, Orazio EN, et al. Prognostic significance of hyperglycemia in acute stroke. Arch Neurol 1985;42:661–3.

134. Baird TA, Parsons MW, Phanh T, et al. Persistent post-stroke hyperglycemia is independently associated with infarct expansion and worse clinical outcome. Stroke 2003;34:2208–14.

135. NICE-SUGAR Investigators. Intensive versus conventional glucose control in critically ill patients. N Engl J Med 2009;360:1283–97.

136. Green DM, O'Phelan KH, Bassin SL, et al. Intensive versus conventional insulin therapy in critically ill neurologic patients. Neurocrit Care 2010;13:299–306.

137. Oddo M, Schmidt JM, Carrera E, et al. Impact of tight glycemic control on cerebral glucose metabolism after severe brain injury: a microdialysis study. Crit Care Med 2008;36:3233–8.

138. Hinchey JA, Shephard T, Furie K, et al. Formal dysphagia screening protocols prevent pneumonia. Stroke 2005;36:1972–6.

139. Martino R, Foley N, Bhogal S, et al. Dysphagia after stroke: incidence, diagnosis, and pulmonary complications. Stroke 2005;36:2756–63.

140. DePippo KL, Holas MA, Reding MJ. Validation of the 3-oz water swallow test for aspiration following stroke. Arch Neurol 1992;49:1259–61.

141. Kelly J, Rudd A, Lewis RR, et al. Venous thromboembolism after acute ischemic stroke: a prospective study using magnetic resonance direct thrombus imaging. Stroke 2004;35:2320–5.

142. Raslan AM, Fields JD, Bhardwaj A. Prophylaxis for venous thrombo-embolism in neurocritical care: a critical appraisal. Neurocrit Care 2010;12:297–309.

143. Mazzone C, Chiodo GF, Sandercock P, et al. Physical methods for preventing deep venous thrombosis in stroke. Cochrane Database Syst Rev 2004;(4):CD0001922.

144. Schirmer CM, Kornbluth J, Heilman CB, et al. Gastrointestinal prophylaxis in neurocritical care. Neurocrit Care 2012;16(1):184–93.

145. Rabinstein AA, Hemphill JC 3rd. Prognosticating after severe, acute brain disease: science, art, and biases. Neurology 2010;74:1086–7.
146. Becker KJ, Baxter AB, Cohen WA, et al. Withdrawal of support in intracerebral hemorrhage may lead to self-fulfilling prophecies. Neurology 2001;56:766–72.

Transient Ischemic Attack
Reviewing the Evolution of the Definition, Diagnosis, Risk Stratification, and Management for the Emergency Physician

Matthew S. Siket, MD, MS[a], Jonathan A. Edlow, MD[b],*

KEYWORDS

- Transient ischemic attack • Emergency medicine • Risk stratification • Diagnosis
- Management

KEY POINTS

- Take a careful history to establish the abrupt onset of symptoms that fit within a particular cerebrovascular territory, which is the cornerstone of making the diagnosis of TIA.
- If the neurologic examination has not completely normalized, treat as a stroke not a TIA.
- All patients diagnosed with a TIA should receive some form of antiplatelet therapy.
- Because approximately 5% of patients with TIA will have a stroke within 48 hours of the TIA, a rapid workup and implementation of treatments are crucial to reducing that stroke risk.
- The only time it is truly safe to discharge patients with TIA is if they do not have an acutely interventional lesion (eg, carotid stenosis or atrial fibrillation). If this workup can be done in the ED or an observation unit, strongly consider inpatient evaluation.

BACKGROUND
Introduction

A transient ischemic attack (TIA) is an episode of reversible neurologic deficit caused by temporary focal central nervous system hypoperfusion. In many cases, the symptoms will resolve by the time patients first see the physician; therefore, the diagnosis requires a careful history. TIA is a medical emergency. TIA and ischemic stroke are parts of the same continuum of acute cerebrovascular syndrome (ACVS) just as angina and acute myocardial infarction are part of the continuum of acute coronary

[a] Department of Emergency Medicine, Harvard Medical School, Massachusetts General Hospital, Boston, MA, USA; [b] Department of Emergency Medicine, Beth Israel Deaconess Medical Center, Harvard Medical School, Boston, MA, USA
* Corresponding author.
E-mail address: jedlow@bidmc.harvard.edu

Emerg Med Clin N Am 30 (2012) 745–770
doi:10.1016/j.emc.2012.05.001
0733-8627/12/$ – see front matter © 2012 Elsevier Inc. All rights reserved.

syndromes. Because patients with TIA in the emergency department (ED) have a high risk for stroke within the next 48 hours, it is imperative for the clinician to recognize this golden opportunity to prevent a disabling stroke, the fourth leading cause of death and highest cause of disability in the United States.[1] This article reviews our conceptual understanding of TIA, its definition, diagnosis, ways to stratify stroke risk, the acute management and disposition in the ED, and the potential future role of diagnostic biomarkers.

History and Definition

The concept of TIA dates back to our earliest understanding of the cerebral vasculature. Sir Thomas Willis, credited with coining the term neurology and describing the vascular circle at the base of the brain that bears his name, is also considered the first to write about warning spells of impending cerebral dysfunction. In 1679 he wrote: "the irradiation of the spirits is wont to be interrupted with little clouds, as it were, scattered here and there, but in the former, the same is forthwith wholly darkened and undergoes total eclipse."[2] Embolic sources were apparent even then because he described "extraneous particles" in the blood as a cause.[2] Similar entities are mentioned in medical texts during the eighteenth and nineteenth century, but it was not until the 1950s when the clinical phenomenon became better recognized. C. Miller Fisher described "prodromal fleeting attacks of paralysis, numbness, tingling, speechlessness, unilateral blindness, or dizziness" often preceded and warned of impending strokes in patients with carotid artery disease.[3] The name TIA emerged in 1965, at the fourth Princeton Cerebrovascular Disease Conference, after extensive discussion at earlier conferences in 1954 and 1956.[4] The classic definition of TIA as "focal cerebral dysfunction of an ischemic nature lasting no longer than 24 hours with a tendency to recur" involves an arbitrary time limit that was agreed on by an ad hoc committee in 1975 and endorsed by the World Health Organization in 1988.[5] This definition persisted for many years despite the knowledge that most TIAs last less than 1 hour. In an era before magnetic resonance imaging (MRI), thrombolytic treatment of ischemic stroke, and a better understanding of the hyperacute risk of stroke following TIA, this older definition sufficed. However, in an era marked by these 3 realities, a plea for a modernized tissue-based rather than time-based definition was formally made in 2002 and eventually endorsed by the American Heart Association/American Stroke Association (AHA/ASA) in 2009.[6] Thus, the current definition of TIA is "a transient episode of neurologic dysfunction caused by focal brain, spinal cord, or retinal ischemia, without acute infarction."[7] Importantly, the element of time is no longer a component of the definition (**Box 1**).

The revised tissue-based definition fragmentized the clinical entities previously referred to as TIA and created a diagnostic dilemma in cases of transient symptoms with imaging evidence of infarction. A source of debate, it remains unresolved whether this is better classified as TIA, ischemic stroke, or a distinct entity unto itself. It has been proposed that transient symptoms with infarction (TSI) should be operationally considered distinct, which is akin to unstable angina in the spectrum of acute coronary syndrome.[8] Collectively, the spectrum of ACVS includes TIA, TSI, and ischemic stroke.

Box 1
Revised definition of TIA endorsed by the AHA/ASA

"A transient episode of neurologic dysfunction caused by focal brain, spinal cord, or retina ischemia, without acute infarction."[7]

Epidemiology

The incidence of TIA in the United States is estimated to be between 200,000 and 500,000, with a prevalence of approximately 5 million people.[9] More than one-third of patients will fail to seek medical attention within the first 24 hours of the event.[10] TIAs are diagnosed in approximately 0.3% of ED visits.[11] Men are more likely than women and African Americans are more likely than Caucasians to experience a TIA.[12,13] TIAs were found to be more common among lower-income individuals and those with fewer years of education in one study.[10] Regardless of ethnicity, gender, or socioeconomic status, TIA incidence increases exponentially with advancing age.[13]

Stroke Risk

Overall, stroke is preceded by a TIA in 12% to 30% of patients and a quarter of these will occur shortly after the TIA.[14,15] For decades, it was clear that the long-term (3–5 years) outcome of ischemic stroke following TIA was approximately 30% to 40%. However, in 2000, new data suggested that much of this risk is front loaded in the first hours to days after the TIA.[16] The risk of stroke is highest within the first 24 hours and decreases steadily thereafter.[17] Roughly 11% of patients that experience a TIA will suffer a disabling stroke within 90 days and, of those, half will do so within the first 48 hours following the TIA.[18] Furthermore, stroke risk has been shown to be dependent on the underlying pathologic condition that caused the TIA. Hemispheric TIA from tight internal carotid artery (ICA) stenosis is associated with the highest risk of stroke (20.0% at 3 months) compared with other causes (5.7%), such as intracranial small vessel disease and cardioembolism.[19]

Causes

TIAs and ischemic strokes share the same list of causes, most commonly, the embolic or thrombotic consequences of atherothrombotic disease. When a vascular lesion is found, approximately 25% are caused by thrombotic or embolic complications of atheroma in large- to medium-sized arteries; 25% by intracranial small vessel disease; 20% by cardioembolism; and 5% from less-common causes, such as arterial dissection and hypercoagulable states.[20] Unfortunately, in one-quarter to one-half of cases, no clear vascular mechanism is found.[21,22] Whether this signifies a lack of sensitivity of routine diagnostic tests or confounding by the presence of TIA mimics remains to be determined.

CLINICAL PRESENTATION

When approaching patients with symptoms suggestive of a TIA, the physician's first objective is to determine whether the described episode is consistent with TIA or not. Misdiagnosis rates among emergency physicians has been reported to be as high as 60%,[23] and discordance among neurologists in the diagnosis of TIA by history is thought to be between 42% and 86%.[24,25] Moreover, one recent study found that agreement in the diagnosis of TIA was low even among stroke-trained neurologists, emphasizing its subjectivity.[26]

Onset is characteristically sudden; gradual or marching progression of symptoms is unusual. Symptom duration is usually brief, with 60% of events lasting less than 1 hour.[27] History should be directed at ascertaining the abruptness of the onset and the duration of the symptoms. Another useful part of the history is to try to distinguish negative symptoms, which suggest ischemia or infarction, from positive symptoms, which suggest migraine or seizure. Negative symptoms include the loss of sensation,

However, only 3% of TTEs in patients with stroke or TIA reveal a cardioembolic source in patients lacking other signs of heart disease.[42] Transesophageal echocardiogram (TEE) is more sensitive for the detection of aortic arch atheroma, patent foramen ovale, atrial septal defect, atrial thrombus, and valvular vegetation but is more time consuming, invasive, and requires sedation. Collectively, TTE or TEE in patients with TIA yields a major source of cardioembolism in 10% of patients and a minor source in 46%.[43] In cryptogenic stroke and TIA, TEE uncovered potentially treatable embolic sources in 61% of patients.[44]

Brain Imaging

The new tissue-based definition of TIA was generated out of a wealth of data showing that 30% to 50% of patients with traditionally defined TIAs have evidence of infarction on MRI.[45–47] Thus, the AHA/ASA currently recommends that all patients with TIA undergo emergent neuroimaging within 24 hours of symptom onset (class I, level B).[47] MRI is the preferred modality if available. MRI with diffusion-weighted imaging (DWI) is far more sensitive to infarction (especially early in its course) than computed tomography (CT) (**Figs. 1 and 2**).[48] Reports on the sensitivity of CT to detect acute infarcts range from 4% to 34%.[49,50] DWI detects areas of restricted diffusion consistent with cytotoxic edema formation in the ischemic brain, making it the clearly superior imaging modality. However, MRI has several restrictions and is contraindicated in approximately 10% of patients.[51,52] Additionally, only 39% of US EDs have 24-hour access to MRI,[53] and only between 5% and 15% of health care providers use MRI as the first-line imaging modality of choice in evaluating TIA.[11,54] Despite its limitations, CT remains the most common neuroimaging study obtained in patients with TIA presenting to the ED, reportedly performed in 56% to 92% of cases.[11,54]

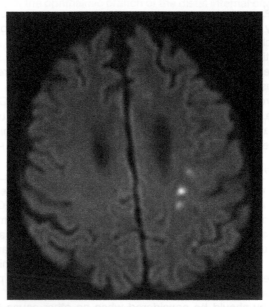

Fig. 1. This diffusion-weighted image reveals multiple punctate foci of restricted diffusion consistent with acute infarction. This patient experienced transient symptoms and had an National Institutes of Health Stroke Scale of zero in the emergency department, indicating transient symptoms with infarction.

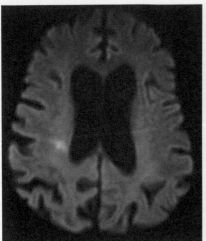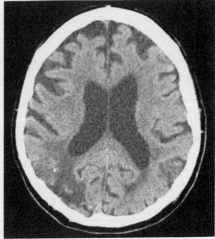

Fig. 2. Computed tomography and diffusion-weighted images from a patient with a prior right parieto-occipital infarct presenting with transient symptoms and found to have an acute infarct in the adjacent territory.

Determining ways to improve the predictive ability of CT for early stroke risk is an area worthy of further research.

Vascular Imaging

Nearly half of the patients with TIA with DWI lesions have stenosis or occlusion of either extracranial or intracranial large arteries, suggesting that vascular imaging is imperative in the acute evaluation of TIA.[55] Presently, routine noninvasive cervicocephalic vessel imaging is recommended by the AHA/ASA as part of the acute evaluation of TIA (class I, level A).[7] This imaging can be performed by ultrasound using carotid duplex and transcranial Doppler (TCD) or with noninvasive CT or MR angiography (MRA), technologies that have largely supplanted the use of traditional catheter-based cerebral angiography. Advantages and disadvantages of each vascular imaging modality are listed in **Table 1**.

Carotid duplex ultrasound detects significant (>50%) stenosis of the extracranial portion of the ICA with sensitivity and specificity of 88% and 76% respectively.[56] Advantages include its low cost, ease of use, widespread availability, and lack of radiation or contrast. The disadvantages include its insensitivity in detecting arterial dissection and complex but nonflow limiting lesions, operator dependence, and the inability to evaluate the intracranial ICA. TCD and transcranial color Doppler ultrasonography can reliably exclude intracranial stenosis in both the anterior and posterior circulation, with a reported negative predictive value of 86%.[57] TCD was easily performed within 4 hours of presentation to a high-volume TIA clinic and was found to be independently predictive of recurrent vascular events.[58]

Contrast-enhanced MRA detects significant supra-aortic extracranial stenosis with a sensitivity between 82% and 92% and specificity between 80% and 97%.[55,59] Unenhanced time-of-flight sequences provide a reasonable option in those to whom gadolinium cannot be safely administered. MRA performs similarly to TCD in excluding intracranial stenosis, with a reported negative predictive value of 91%.[57]

CT angiography (CTA) is widely available in most EDs and can be performed at the time of the initial unenhanced CT, adding only a few minutes to the total scan

Table 1
Comparison of NPV for various vascular imaging modalities in excluding carotid stenosis greater than 50%

Test	NPV (%)	Advantages	Disadvantages
Duplex US	91[56]	Low cost No IV contrast	Does not visualize intracranial portion of ICA Insensitive for dissection 24-hour availability variable Can miss an ulcerated, nonobstructive plaque
CTA	97[60]	Easily obtainable and widely available Provides detailed images of cervical and cerebral vessels Sensitive for dissection	Additional radiation exposure Requires IV contrast Some bone averaging at skull base
MRA	99[59]	Provides detailed images of cervical and cerebral vessels TOF sequences can obviate contrast if contraindicated	Expensive Time consuming Contraindicated in those with indwelling pacemakers, implants, and so forth ED availability limited

Abbreviations: CTA, CT angiography; IV, intravenous; NPV, negative predictive value; TOF, time of flight; US, ultrasound.

time (**Fig. 3**). It has been reported to achieve a 97% negative predictive value for excluding significant (50%–99%) ICA stenosis compared with traditional angiography.[60] Moreover, CTA performed on 64-slice CT scanners has been shown to provide near equivalent diagnostic information to digital subtraction angiography while imaging the cerebral vasculature with one fixed dose of contrast.[61] Intracranial arterial occlusion on CTA has been shown to be an independent predictor of poor outcome

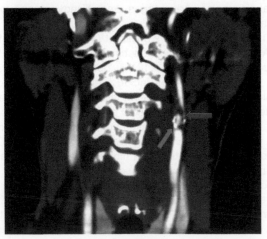

Fig. 3. Coronal computed tomography angiography image from a patient with critical internal carotid artery stenosis (*red arrow*) and calcified atherosclerotic plaque (*green arrow*).

after stroke and TIA, and most recently CT/CTA abnormalities were found to be equivalent in predicting 90-day stroke recurrence after TIA and minor stroke.[62–64] CTA also reliably excludes cervical vessel dissection. Limitations include the need for intravenous contrast and the additional radiation, which has been shown to be between double and triple the dose of a standard CT brain (1.7–2.7 mSv to 4.7–5.4 mSv for CT head and neck).[65]

The role of perfusion imaging has been explored in TIA but is currently not considered part of routine care. Studies have shown that MR perfusion weighted imaging (PWI) abnormalities are present in 30% to 40% of patients with TIA, and isolated perfusion abnormalities in an otherwise normal MRI are present in 14% to 16% of cases.[66–69] Furthermore, CT perfusion has recently been shown to detect abnormalities in one-third of the patients with TIA, which was predictive of in-hospital adverse events, including recurrent TIA and stroke, and was independent of DWI lesions or other traditional risk-stratification tools.[70] The current opinion in the neurology community supports PWI as a complimentary tool to DWI in the evaluation of TIA, and at least one study has shown perfusion abnormalities to be predictive of ischemic recurrence at 1 week.[71,72]

RISK PREDICTION

There have been numerous attempts over the past 20 years to create a validated risk-stratification tool that is easy to apply and provides clinicians with a realistic estimate of stroke risk after TIA. The first seems to be the Stroke Prognosis Instrument published by Kernan and colleagues[73] in 1991. This tool was followed by Hankey and colleagues[74] in 1992, then the California Score in 2000,[16] and the ABCD score in 2005.[75] The ABCD2 score published in 2007 represents the combined efforts of the authors of the California and ABCD scores and has demonstrated the best discriminative predictive ability. It stratifies patients as low, moderate, or high risk of stroke following TIA at 2, 7, and 90 days.[76] **Table 2** lists the ABCD2 score and its predictive ability at 2, 7, and 90 days compared with the California and ABCD scores in **Table 3**.

Although the ABCD2 score has raised awareness of the urgency of TIA evaluation in the ED, little consensus exists as to its proper implementation. Since its original publication, several external validation studies have shown mixed results.[77–89] Some have argued that the value of the ABCD2 score is in its discriminative ability to differentiate true transient ischemic events from mimics.[81] Others have suggested that the ABCD2 score does not predict who will have an infarct in the short-term but rather in which patients the infarct is likely to be severe and disabling.[80]

Table 2 The ABCD2 score	
	Points
A = Age >60 y	1
B = Blood pressure >140/90	1
C = Clinical features: unilateral weakness (2), speech difficulty without weakness (1)	2
D = Duration: >60 min (2), 10–59 min (1), <10 min (0)	2
D = Diabetes	1
Total	7

Data from Johnston SC, Rothwell PM, Nguyen-Huynh MN, et al. Validation and refinement of scores to predict very early stroke risk after transient ischaemic attack. Lancet 2007;369:283–92.

Table 5				
Seven-day stroke risk by imaging modality and ABCD2 score				
Imaging Modality	Infarction Present?	ABCD2 Score	7-Day Stroke Risk (%)	Upper Limit 95% CI
CT	No	0–3	0.9	2.6
		4–5	3.0	4.9
		6–7	7.3	12.2
	Yes	0–3	3.9	11.5
		4–5	12.9	19.6
		6–7	21.0	33.6
MRI	No	0–3	0.1	0.5
		4–5	0.7	1.4
		6–7	0.4	2.1
	Yes	0–3	1.8	4.6
		4–5	7.5	10.4
		6–7	12.5	18.6

Abbreviation: CI, confidence interval.
Data from Giles MF, Albers GW, Amarenco P, et al. Early stroke risk and ABCD2 score performance in tissue- versus time-defined TIA. Neurology 2011;77:1222–8.

have been developed to ease the determination of stroke cause and improve inter-rater agreement.[94–96] A Web-based recurrence risk estimator score was developed specifically for TSI because these individuals have been shown to be at the highest risk of stroke in the short-term.[97,98]

The AHA/ASA and National Institutes for Health and Clinical Excellence (NICE) guidelines now incorporate the ABCD2 score and imaging findings into acute management and disposition recommendations in TIA.[7,99] Regardless of whether a newer mechanism-driven or imaging-enhanced risk-prediction tool is used, there is general consensus that a complete etiologic workup should be performed as urgently as possible. The distinction between accurate risk stratification and completing the etiologic workup up front is blurred, calling into question where to draw the line in the ED. It has been suggested elsewhere, and remains the opinion of these authors, that taking a work-up-everybody policy by performing as much of an etiologic workup in the ED as logistically possible is the best way to ensure that patients receive optimal care during the period of highest stroke risk.[90] This policy could mean hospitalizing patients or performing the evaluation in the ED. If this is not logistically feasible in a given location, then the physician should consider using the ABCD2 score and organize the workup as per the AHA 2009 guidelines.[7]

MANAGEMENT
General Considerations

The primary goals in patients with TIA and TSI are to optimize cerebral perfusion to the ischemic tissue and to prevent a subsequent more disabling stroke. Positioning the patient with the head of the bed flat has been shown (by TCD) to increase cerebral perfusion by 20% compared with a 30° incline.[100] This simple step should be done routinely unless contraindicated. As in ischemic stroke, it is generally a good idea to maintain euvolemia, and all patients with TIA should have intravenous access while in the ED. Conflicting data exist as to the utility of supplementary oxygen in patients with cerebral ischemia but is generally not recommended unless patients are hypoxic.[101,102]

Antihypertensive Treatment

Permissive hypertension is the strategy of avoiding aggressive treatment of elevated blood pressure in the acute setting. It is thought that patients with cerebral ischemia may have impaired cerebral autoregulation and require higher mean arterial pressures to maximize the perfusion of collateral vessels. Current AHA/ASA consensus panel recommends that emergency administration of antihypertensives be withheld unless blood pressure is greater than 220/120 mm Hg.[103] Multiple studies have demonstrated worse outcomes after stroke in those treated acutely with blood-pressure lowering agents.[104,105] Unlike stroke, patients with TIA are probably less likely to experience drops in cerebral perfusion pressure; to date, outpatient oral antihypertensive treatment initiated during the initial evaluation has not been associated with worsened outcomes.[106,107] Currently, the AHA/ASA recommends initiating antihypertensive medications in patients who remain stable *beyond the first 24 hours* following a TIA or stroke.[108] Therefore, prescribing antihypertensive medication is not generally an ED issue, unless one is discharging a patient from an ED-based observation unit. The target blood pressure after the first 24 hours remains to be determined, but a reduction of 10/5 mm Hg or normalization to less than 120/80 using a diuretic or angiotensin-converting enzyme inhibitor is supported.[108]

Antiplatelet Therapy

Absent a specific contraindication or a cardioembolic source that necessitates full anticoagulation, every patient with TIA should receive antiplatelet therapy.

The Food and Drug Administration has approved 4 antiplatelet agents for the prevention of vascular events following TIA or stroke. These agents include aspirin, aspirin/dipyridamole combination, clopidogrel, and ticlopidine, which have collectively demonstrated an average reduction of the relative risk of stroke, myocardial infarction, or death of 22%.[109] Clopidogrel and aspirin/dipyridamole have demonstrated superiority to aspirin alone, and a head-to-head trial comparing these 2 agents showed similar efficacy and safety profiles.[22,110] To date, combination therapy with aspirin and clopidogrel has not demonstrated benefit over clopidogrel or aspirin alone but has shown an increase in bleeding complications and is not routinely recommended.[111-113] In some situations in which clopidogrel is indicated for another reason (such as coronary artery disease), aspirin plus clopidogrel may be indicated. Ticlopidine is rarely used because of its side-effect profile.

Anticoagulation

For patients with TIA or stroke that is thought to be caused by atrial fibrillation, anticoagulation with warfarin is advised (target international normalized ratio [INR] of 2.5; range 2–3; AHA/ASA class I; level A recommendation).[108] Dabigatran is a direct thrombin inhibitor that has demonstrated noninferiority to warfarin in preventing stroke in patients with atrial fibrillation and is a reasonable alternative, although no known reversal agent exists to date.[114] If oral anticoagulants are contraindicated, aspirin alone is recommended. See **Tables 6** and **7** for pharmacologic recommendations by TIA cause and dosing.

Endovascular Treatment of Cervical Carotid Stenosis

In patients with imaging evidence of severe (>70%) carotid stenosis, carotid endarterectomy (CEA) significantly reduces stroke risk.[115] Overall stroke risk reduction in these patients is 10% to 15% and seems to be more beneficial in older patients (aged >75 years). A similar benefit seems to exist in patients with 50% to 70% stenosis and the

Table 6
Management recommendations by TIA or minor stroke cause

Cause	Incidence (%)	Management	
Large artery atherosclerosis	~25	Antiplatelet therapy, and if carotid stenosis >50%, evaluation for endarterectomy to be performed preferably within 2 wk	Initiate statin therapy, optimization of comorbidities (such as hypertension and diabetes), and risk factor modification
Small vessel disease	~25	Antiplatelet therapy	
Cardioembolic	~20	Anticoagulation	
Arterial dissection	~5	Antiplatelet therapy or anticoagulation for 3–6 mo	
Hypercoagulable state and inherited thrombophilias		Hematologic workup and condition-specific anticoagulation or antiplatelet therapy	
Cryptogenic or unknown	~25	Antiplatelet therapy	

benefit is greatest if performed within 2 weeks of the sentinel event.[115] Carotid angioplasty and stenting is considered a reasonable alternative to CEA, particularly in those considered at high risk for surgical complications.[108] Decisions about which method of opening the carotids are beyond the scope of emergency medicine practice.

Table 7
Commonly used medications for stroke prevention after TIA

Therapy	Agent	Dose	Indication
Antiplatelet	Aspirin	160–325 mg/d acutely, then 81 mg/d	All acute TIA
	Aspirin/ dipyridamole combination	Aspirin 25 mg + extended- release dipyridamole 200 mg/d	Stroke prevention after TIA: better than aspirin alone and equivalent to clopidogrel
	Clopidogrel	300 mg/d acutely, then 75 mg/d	Stroke prevention in patients with aspirin allergy
Anticoagulation	Heparin	Parenteral to target PTT	Stuttering TIA or known cardioembolic source or severe large vessel stenosis
	Warfarin	Dose to target INR of 2–3	TIA caused by atrial fibrillation
	Dabigatran	150 mg twice daily (renal dose is 75 mg twice daily)	TIA caused by atrial fibrillation

Abbreviation: PTT, partial thromboplastin time.
Data from Cucchiara B, Kasner SE. In the clinic: transient ischemic attack. Ann Intern Med 2011;154:ITC11-15 [quiz: ITC1–16].

Lipid Modification

Lowering cholesterol with statins has been shown to reduce the risk of vascular events in patients with TIA and stroke.[116] Statins are thought to stabilize atherosclerotic plaques; decrease the intimal-medial thickness of the carotids; and promote antioxidant, antiinflammatory, and antiplatelet effects.[22] The current AHA/ASA recommendation is to initiate statins after TIA or stroke for patients with an low-density lipoprotein (LDL) greater than 100 mg/dL with a target goal of an LDL level of less than 70 mg/dL.[108]

Risk-Factor Modification

Other independent risk factors associated with stroke include cigarette smoking and heavy alcohol consumption. Obese (body mass index >30 kg/m^3) patients should be counseled on weight-reduction strategies, although to date no study has demonstrated that weight loss reduces stroke risk. Moderate physical activity has been shown to reduce stroke risk by 20%.[117]

Special Circumstances

For patients with TIA or stroke secondary to cervical arterial dissection, the AHA/ASA currently recommends antithrombotic treatment for 3 to 6 months. There is no clear consensus whether anticoagulation or antiplatelet therapy is superior; therapy should be individualized. Dissections generally heal with time, but if recurrent cerebral ischemic events occur, endovascular stenting may be considered. For patients with documented patent foramen ovale, the optimal treatment remains in question and is the subject of ongoing investigation. The role of the emergency physician in these cases will be to facilitate appropriate cardiology and neurology referral, although initiating antiplatelet therapy is reasonable with specialty consultation.[108] If infective endocarditis is the suspected source of emboli, blood cultures, early antiinfective treatment, and cardiology consultation is indicated.[118]

Thrombolysis

Rapidly improving symptoms and minor neurologic deficits are considered contraindications to thrombolytic administration, so their use in TIA is not recommended. However, because the risk of stroke following TIA is frontloaded and highest within the ensuing 48 hours, access to recombinant tissue plasminogen activator (rt-PA) is imperative. This point is particularly true in patients with stuttering or crescendo TIAs who experience frequent episodes and carry a more ominous prognosis in the short term. In terms of the time window, one starts the clock from the time when patients were last completely normal; that is, for patients with waxing and waning symptoms, the last time they were totally normal would count for the time window. Patients and caretakers should be cautioned to return immediately if symptoms return so that thrombolysis can be given if indicated. Patients should also be educated about time windows for therapy and how to access 911 to rapidly get to a stroke center.

DISPOSITION

Determining which patients to admit to the hospital versus observe in an observation unit or discharge with rapid follow-up is a source of uncertainty and frustration for many emergency physicians. Factors likely to contribute to varying admission thresholds include the ease of access to follow-up testing and neurology consultation, inpatient bed availability, patient expectations, and medicolegal concerns.

Some have advocated for admission policies based on the ABCD2 score. In reviewing the cohorts used to create and validate the ABCD2 score, a policy limited to

129. Rothwell PM, Giles MF, Chandratheva A, et al. Effect of urgent treatment of transient ischaemic attack and minor stroke on early recurrent stroke (EXPRESS study): a prospective population-based sequential comparison. Lancet 2007; 370:1432–42.

130. Whiteley W, Tseng MC, Sandercock P. Blood biomarkers in the diagnosis of ischemic stroke: a systematic review. Stroke 2008;39:2902–9.

131. Corso G, Bottacchi E, Brusa A, et al. Blood C-reactive protein concentration with ABCD^2 is a better prognostic tool than ABCD^2 alone. Cerebrovasc Dis 2011;32: 97–105.

132. Katan M, Nigro N, Flurl F, et al. Stress hormones predict cerebrovascular re-events after transient ischemic attacks. Neurology 2011;76:563–6.

133. Cucchiara BL, Messe SR, Sansing L, et al. Lipoprotein-associated phospholipase A2 and C-reactive protein for risk-stratification of patients with TIA. Stroke 2009;40:2332–6.

134. Montaner J, Perea-Gainza M, Delgado P, et al. Etiologic diagnosis of ischemic stroke subtypes with plasma biomarkers. Stroke 2008;39:2280–7.

135. Zhan X, Jickling GC, Tian Y, et al. Transient ischemic attacks characterized by RNA profiles in blood. Neurology 2011;77:1718–24.

136. Montaner J, Mendioroz M, Ribo M, et al. A panel of biomarkers including caspase-3 and D-dimer may differentiate acute stroke from stroke-mimicking conditions in the emergency department. J Intern Med 2011;270:166–74.

Intracranial Hemorrhage

J. Alfredo Caceres, MD[a], Joshua N. Goldstein, MD, PhD[b,c],*

KEYWORDS

- Intracranial hemorrhage • Acute stroke • Intracerebral hemorrhage
- Subarachnoid hemorrhage

KEY POINTS

- Intracerebral hemorrhage is the most devastating form of stroke, with high mortality and severe disability among survivors.
- While no single therapy has been demonstrated to improve outcome, there is evidence that high quality supportive care can provide substantial benefit.
- National evidence-based guidelines are available to guide management for both intracerebral hemorrhage and subarachnoid hemorrhage.
- Ruptured aneurysms are best managed by teams with experience in both surgical and endovascular techniques.

INTRODUCTION

Intracranial hemorrhage refers to any bleeding within the intracranial vault, including the brain parenchyma and surrounding meningeal spaces. This article focuses on the acute diagnosis and management of primary nontraumatic intracerebral hemorrhage (ICH) and subarachnoid hemorrhage (SAH) in emergency departments (EDs).

INTRACEREBRAL HEMORRHAGE

ICH is a devastating disease. The overall incidence of spontaneous ICH worldwide is 24.6 per 100,000 person-years with approximately 40,000 to 67,000 cases per year in the United States.[1–3] The 30-day mortality rate ranges from 35% to 52% with only 20% of survivors expected to have full functional recovery at 6 months.[3] Approximately half of this mortality occurs within the first 24 hours,[4] highlighting the critical importance of early and effective treatment in EDs.

Risk Factors

A recent population-based meta-analysis showed that risk factors for ICH include male gender, older age, and Asian ethnicity.[1,5] ICH is twice as frequent in low-income to

[a] Department of Neurology, Massachusetts General Hospital, Suite 3B, Zero Emerson Place, Boston, MA 01940, USA; [b] Harvard Medical School, 25 Shattuck Street, Boston, MA 02115, USA; [c] Department of Emergency Medicine, Massachusetts General Hospital, Suite 3B, Zero Emersion place, Boston, MA 01940, USA
* Corresponding author.
E-mail address: jgoldstein@partners.org

Emerg Med Clin N Am 30 (2012) 771–794
http://dx.doi.org/10.1016/j.emc.2012.06.003
0733-8627/12/$ – see front matter © 2012 Elsevier Inc. All rights reserved.

emed.theclinics.com

middle-income countries compared with high-income countries.[5] In the United States, several studies have shown that the incidence of ICH is greater in African Americans and Hispanics than in whites.[6–8]

The most important risk factors for ICH include hypertension (HTN) and cerebral amyloid angiopathy (CAA). HTN-related ICH is more likely to occur in deep structures,[9] and the risk of ICH increases with increasing blood pressure (BP) values.[10] CAA tends to occur in association with advanced age, and CAA-related ICH tends to occur in lobar regions.[11]

Other risk factors for ICH include

1. Alcohol intake: this risk seems dose-dependent, with a higher risk of ICH among those with a higher daily alcohol intake.[10] Acute changes in BP during ingestion and withdrawal, effects on platelet function and coagulation, and dysfunction of the vascular endothelium may account for this risk.[12]
2. Cholesterol: low levels of total serum cholesterol are risk factors for ICH (in contrast to ischemic stroke, for which high cholesterol levels are a risk).[13]
3. Genetics: the gene most strongly associated with ICH is the apolipoprotein E gene and its ε2 and ε4 alleles.[14] The presence of the ε2 allele was recently also linked to hematoma expansion.[15]
4. Anticoagulation: oral anticoagulants are widely used as prophylaxis in patients with atrial fibrillation and other cardiovascular and prothrombotic states. The annual risk of ICH in patients taking warfarin ranges from 0.3% to 1.0% per patient-year, with a significantly increased risk when the international normalized ratio (INR) is greater than 3.5.[16]
5. Drug abuse: sympathomimetic drugs, such as cocaine, are risk factors for ICH, and patients actively using cocaine at the time of their ICH have significantly more severe presentations and worse outcomes.[17]

Pathophysiology

Primary ICH is typically a manifestation of underlying small vessel disease. First, long-standing HTN leads to hypertensive vasculopathy, causing microscopic degenerative changes in the walls of small-to-medium penetrating vessels, which is known as lipohyalinosis.[18] Second, CAA is characterized by the deposition of amyloid-β peptide in the walls of small leptomeningeal and cortical vessels.[19] Although the underlying mechanism leading to the accumulation of amyloid is still unknown, the final consequences are degenerative changes in the vessel wall characterized by the loss of smooth muscle cells, wall thickening, luminal narrowing, microaneurysm formation, and microhemorrhages.[20]

After initial vessel rupture, the hematoma causes direct mechanical injury to the brain parenchyma. Perihematomal edema develops within the first 3 hours from symptom onset and peaks between 10 and 20 days.[21] Next, blood and plasma products mediate secondary injury processes, including an inflammatory response, activation of the coagulation cascade, and iron deposition from hemoglobin degradation.[21] Finally, the hematoma can continue to expand in up to 38% of patients during the first 24 hours.[22]

Clinical Presentation and Diagnosis

The acute presentation of ICH can be difficult to distinguish from ischemic stroke. Symptoms may include headache, nausea, seizures, and focal or generalized neurologic symptoms. Findings, such as coma, headache, vomiting, seizures, neck stiffness, and raised diastolic BP, increase the likelihood of ICH compared with ischemic stroke, but only neuroimaging can provide a definitive diagnosis.[23]

Neuroimaging

Noncontrast CT

Noncontrast CT is the most rapid and readily available tool for the diagnosis of ICH[24] and remains the most commonly used technique in the ED. Besides providing the definitive diagnosis, CT may also show basic characteristics of the hematoma, such as hematoma location, extension to the ventricular system, presence of surrounding edema, development of mass effect, and midline shift.

A quick estimation of the hematoma volume can be rapidly performed in an ED with the validated ABC/2 technique (**Fig. 1**).[25] The steps to follow using this technique are

- The CT slice with the largest area of hemorrhage is selected.
- A is the largest hemorrhage diameter on the selected slice (in centimeters [cm]).
- B is the largest diameter perpendicular to A on the same slice.
- C is the approximate number of slices in which the hemorrhage is seen multiplied by the slice thickness (often 0.5-cm slices).
- A, B, and C are multiplied and the product divided by 2.

CT angiography

CT angiography (CTA) is gaining increasing acceptance as a diagnostic tool in the acute setting.[26] It is the most widely available, noninvasive technique for ruling out vascular abnormalities as secondary causes of ICH. The risk of acute nephropathy, if any, is likely low.[27] Up to 15% of patients with ICH show an underlying vascular etiology on CTA, potentially changing acute management.[28] Finally, contrast extravasation seen on CTA images, also known as a spot sign (**Fig. 2**), is thought to represent ongoing bleeding and seems to mark those patients at highest risk of hematoma expansion and with poor outcome and mortality.[29–32]

MRI

MRI is equivalent to CT for the detection of acute ICH.[33] The imaging characteristics of ICH vary with time as the hemoglobin passes through different stages during the

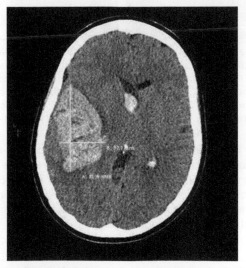

Fig. 1. ABC/2 technique. (*From* Li N, Wang Y, Wang W, et al. Contrast extravasation on computed tomography angiography predicts clinical outcome in primary intracerebral hemorrhage. Stroke 2011;42:3441–6; with permission.)

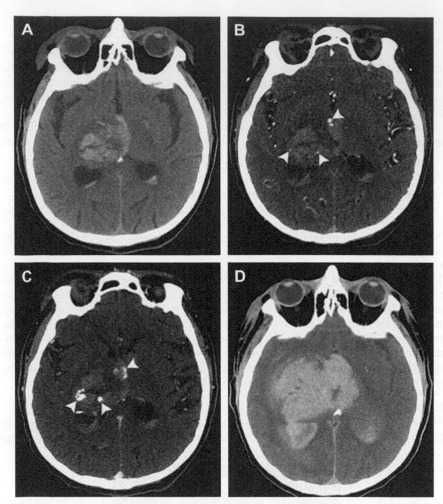

Fig. 2. CT and CTA of acute ICH. (*A*) Noncontrast CT shows a right thalamic ICH (24 mL) with associated IVH (6 mL). (*B*) CTA demonstrates 3 foci of contrast (spot signs) within the ICH (*arrowheads*) (*C*). Delayed CTA shows increased volume and changed morphology of the spot signs (*arrowheads*). (*D*) Noncontrast CT after 8 hours demonstrates expansion of the ICH (94 mL) and IVH (82 mL). (*From* Kidwell CS, Chalela JA, Saver JL, et al. Comparison of MRI and CT for detection of acute intracerebral hemorrhage. JAMA 2004;292[15]:1823–30; with permission.)

pathologic process. In the acute phase, gradient-recalled-echo imaging techniques with T2* weighting are the best option to detect the presence of ICH.[34] MRI can also detect underlying secondary causes of ICH, such as tumor and hemorrhagic transformation of ischemic stroke. Finally, for patients with poor kidney function or contrast allergies, the cerebral vasculature can be analyzed without contrast using time-of-flight magnetic resonance angiography.[35]

Acute Management

Airway
Patients with ICH are often unable to protect the airway. Endotracheal intubation may be necessary but this decision should be balanced against the risk of losing the

neurologic examination. Rapid sequence intubation is typically the preferred approach in the acute setting. Pretreatment with lidocaine may be considered because it may blunt a rise in intracranial pressure (ICP) associated with intubation. Paralytic agents include succinylcholine, rocuronium, and vecuronium, and, for postintubation sedation, propofol is a reasonable choice, given its short half-life.[36,37]

Blood pressure management

Elevated BP is common in the acute setting after an ICH, and higher BP levels are associated with hematoma expansion and poor prognosis. It is not clear, however, that reducing BP improves outcomes.[38] Although lowering BP may reduce the risk of expansion, it may theoretically also reduce cerebral perfusion. One randomized clinical trial found that lowering systolic BP (SBP) to 140 mm Hg compared with 180 mm Hg reduced the risk of hematoma expansion but had no effect on outcomes.[39] A second trial found that rapid BP lowering using intravenous nicardipine seems safe but again showed no difference in outcomes.[40] Several clinical trials are currently ongoing to address this issue.[41–43]

Until these trials clarify the role of BP management on hematoma expansion, expert guidelines from the American Heart Association/American Stroke Association (AHA/ASA) recommend BP treatment (**Box 1**).[38] The European Stroke Initiative (EUSI) guidelines are similar (**Table 1**).[44]

In choosing medications to manage HTN, intravenous antihypertensives with short half-lives should be considered as first-line therapy. The AHA recommends considering IV labetalol, nicardipine, esmolol, enalapril, hydralazine, sodium nitroprusside, or nitroglycerin.[38] The EUSI recommends IV labetalol, urapidil, sodium nitroprusside, nitroglycerin, or captopril.[44]

Hemostatic therapy

It is tempting to consider that in a patient with ICH, acute hemostatic therapy will provide benefit. One phase III randomized trial in patients with no underlying coagulopathy found no clinical benefit from this approach.[45] As a result, current approaches to hemostasis are focused on correcting any underlying coagulopathies.

Oral anticoagulation The most common class of agent used for oral anticoagulation is warfarin. Many investigators believe that early action to rapidly correct the coagulopathy may prevent continued bleeding.[46] Several therapeutic options are available for warfarin reversal.

Box 1
Recommended guidelines from the AHA/ASA for treating elevated BP in spontaneous ICH

1. If SBP is >200 mm Hg or mean arterial pressure (MAP) is >150 mm Hg, then consider aggressive reduction of BP with continuous intravenous infusion, with frequent BP monitoring every 5 minutes.

2. If SBP is >180 mm Hg or MAP is >130 mm Hg and there is the possibility of elevated ICP, then consider monitoring ICP and reducing BP using intermittent or continuous intravenous medications while maintaining a cerebral perfusion pressure (CPP) ≥60 mm Hg.

3. If SBP is >180 mm Hg or MAP is >130 mm Hg and there is no evidence of elevated ICP, then consider a modest reduction of BP (eg, MAP of 110 mm Hg or target BP of 160/90 mm Hg) using intermittent or continuous intravenous medications to control BP and clinically re-examine the patient every 15 minutes.

Adapted from Morgenstern LB, Hemphill JC III, Anderson C, et al. Guidelines for the management of spontaneous intracerebral hemorrhage. Stroke 2010;41(9):2108–29; with permission.

those patients receiving fever control as part of a multidisciplinary approach.[72] Those with fever should undergo a thorough investigation to find a fever source if possible.[38]

Anemia

The presence of anemia is common in patients with ICH. It is present in up to 25% of cases at admission and is associated with larger hematoma volumes.[73] It also frequently develops during hospital stay.[74] Although current guidelines do not address this issue, a recent study found that packed red blood cell transfusion in these patients was associated with improved survival at 30 days.[74] Therefore, transfusion can be considered in such patients, although the ideal target hemoglobin level has not been determined.

Antiepileptics

Patients with ICH are at an increased risk of developing seizures; however, most of these events are subclinical electroencephalographic findings. Seizures are more common in lobar ICH and during the first 72 hours after admission.[75–77] The majority of patients develop a single episode of seizure during hospitalization, suggesting that those episodes are related to the pathophysiologic processes that occur early after an ICH.[77] The use of prophylactic antiepileptic drugs (AEDs) in patients with ICH is a common practice, although it is not clear that the presence of seizures and/or the use of prophylactic AEDs affects short-term or long-term outcome.[78,79] Some studies have reported an association between AEDs and worse outcome, although these patients were disproportionately exposed to phenytoin as the AED of choice.[80,81]

Currently, the AHA/ASA recommends that AEDs should not be used routinely in patients with ICH. The only clear indications are the presence of clinical seizures or electrographic seizures in patients with a change in mental status. They also suggest that the use of continuous electroencephalography monitoring should be considered in those patients with depressed mental status out of proportion to the degree of brain injury.[38]

Surgical Interventions

External ventricular drain placement

As described previously, some patients may benefit from ICP monitoring. External ventricular drain placement not only provides the ability to monitor ICP but also has the advantage of allowing therapeutic drainage of the cerebrospinal fluid (CSF), which is valuable in patients with hydrocephalus.[82] The AHA recommends that ICP monitoring and treatment be considered in patients with a GCS score less than or equal to 8, those with clinical evidence of transtentorial herniation, or those with significant IVH or hydrocephalus.[38] The EUSI recommends considering continuous ICP monitoring in patients who need mechanical ventilation and recommends medical treatment of elevated ICP if clinical deterioration is related to increasing edema.[44]

Intraventricular thrombolysis

IVH occurs when ICH extends into the ventricles. It occurs in approximately 45% of ICH, more frequently in large and deeply located (caudate nucleus and thalamus) hemorrhages.[83] The presence and the volume of IVH are correlated with poor prognosis in patients with ICH.[84] Although evacuation of an intraventricular clot is currently not routinely recommended, a recent study comparing the use of intraventricular recombinant tissue plasminogen activator (rtPA) to placebo not only showed that the use of rtPA was feasible and safe but also showed a significantly greater rate of blood clot resolution.[85] In addition, a recent meta-analysis found that adding intraventricular fibrinolysis to external ventricular drain placement is associated with better functional outcome,[86] although no prospective randomized trial has evaluated this. The Clot Lysis: Evaluating Accelerated Resolution of Intraventricular Hemorrhage (CLEAR III) study, an ongoing phase III randomized clinical trial, was designed to compare the effect on clinical outcome of the intraventricular use of rtPA compared with placebo (ClinicalTrials.gov [NCT00784134]).

Hematoma evacuation

The role of surgical evacuation is to decrease mass effect related to the presence of blood as well as to minimize secondary injury. The only clear recommendation for immediate surgical intervention is in patients with cerebellar hemorrhages with neurologic deterioration, brainstem compression, and/or hydrocephalus from ventricular obstruction.[38] For these patients, emergency neurosurgical consultation should be obtained. It is less clear, however, whether patients with supratentorial ICH will benefit. One large phase III clinical trial, Surgical Treatment for Intracerebral Hemorrhage (STICH), compared early hematoma evacuation with initial conservative treatment of patients with spontaneous supratentorial ICH.[87] This study showed no difference in outcome, suggesting that surgical evacuation provided no benefit. A subsequent subgroup analysis, however, raised the possibility that those with hematomas less than or equal to 1 cm from the cortical surface (which are more easily accessible) might receive benefit.[87] This possibility is being evaluated in the ongoing STICH II trial.[88] The theoretic idea that hyperacute evacuation of the hematoma would be beneficial was not borne out when a study evaluating the effect of surgery within 4 hours was stopped due to a high rate of rebleeding.[89]

Minimally invasive surgery

The development of less-invasive surgical techniques may decrease the risk of surgical complications. These techniques are showing promising results, particularly in deep hemorrhages where conventional surgery showed no benefit in the past.[90] Minimally invasive stereotactic puncture is reported safe and feasible and may lead to better long-term outcome and fewer complications when compared with conventional craniotomy[91] and conventional medical treatment.[92,93]

Prognosis

Multiple grading scores exist that allow for evidence-based risk stratification in the acute phase. First, the ICH score predicts 30-day mortality using features, such as age, ICH volume, and the presence of IVH, with higher score associated with worse outcome (**Table 2**).[94] Second, the FUNC (functional outcome risk stratification) score predicts functional independence rather than mortality at 90 days (**Table 3**).[95] The higher the FUNC score, the greater the chance of the patient recovering functional independence.

There are some data that poor prognosis can lead to self-fulfilling prophecies of early death. Limiting care via early do-not-resuscitate (DNR) orders, withdrawal of care, or deferral of other life-sustaining interventions is independently associated with both short-term and long-term mortality after ICH, after controlling for clinical markers of disease severity, even in patients who do not specifically require defibrillation.[96] As such, new DNR orders or withdrawal of care is generally not recommended in the ED. The AHA recommends aggressive full care early after ICH onset with postponement of new DNR orders until at least the second full day of hospitalization.[38]

SUBARACHNOID HEMORRHAGE

SAH is defined by the extravasation of blood into the subarachnoid space. The most common cause of SAH is trauma; among nontraumatic cases, rupture of an

Table 2
The ICH Score

Component	ICH Score Points
GCS score	
3–4	2
5–12	1
13–15	0
ICH volume (cm³)	
≥30	1
<30	0
IVH	
Yes	1
No	0
Infratentorial origin of ICH	
Yes	1
No	0
Age (y)	
≥80	1
<80	0

Data from Hemphill JC III, Bonovich DC, Besmertis L, et al. The ICH score: a simple, reliable grading scale for intracerebral hemorrhage. Stroke 2001;32(4):891–7.

Table 3
The FUNC Score

Component	FUNC Score Points
ICH volume (cm³)	
<30	4
30–60	2
>60	0
Age (y)	
<70	2
70–79	1
≥80	0
ICH location	
Lobar	2
Deep	1
Infratentorial	0
GCS score	
≥9	2
≤8	0
Pre-ICH cognitive impairment	
No	1
Yes	0
Total FUNC score	0–11

Data from Rost NS, Smith EE, Chang Y, et al. Prediction of functional outcome in patients with primary intracerebral hemorrhage: the FUNC score. Stroke 2008;39(8):2304–9.

intracranial aneurysm is the leading cause, representing up to 85% of cases. This review focuses on aneurysmal SAH.

Epidemiology

The overall incidence of SAH is between 9 and 20 per 100,000 person-years. SAH is more frequent in women, and the mean age of presentation is 55 years.[97,98] In the United States, the number of cases of SAH is 30,000 per year.[99]

Risk Factors and Prognosis

Major risk factors associated with SAH are current and former history of smoking, HTN, and excessive alcohol intake.[100] Although one-third of cases can be attributed to a current smoking status, this risk seems to rapidly disappear after a few years of smoking cessation.[101] Cocaine use is also associated with SAH, and patients taking cocaine tend to be younger and have a worse outcome.[102,103] First-degree family history as well as some genetic conditions, including autosomal dominant polycystic kidney disease, Marfan syndrome, and Ehlers-Danlos syndrome, are also associated with an increased risk of SAH.[104]

A recent meta-analysis reported that in a population without comorbidities, the prevalence of unruptured intracranial aneurysms is 3.2%.[105] Only a small percentage of these unruptured intracranial aneurysms rupture and cause an SAH. The risk of rupture is increased in cases of previous history of SAH, age older than 60, female gender, and Japanese or Finnish descent. In addition, the risk is greater for aneurysms greater than 10 mm and those located in the posterior circulation.[106–108]

The introduction of surgical treatment options improved the prognosis of patients with SAH.[109] In a retrospective analysis before the introduction of endovascular treatment of SAH, the most important factors predicting poor outcome at 3 months were increasing age, worse admission grade on the World Federation of Neurological Surgeons (WFNS) grading scale (**Table 4**), the development of cerebral infarction, and symptomatic vasospasm. Other factors included greater clot thickness on admission CT scan, aneurysm rupture within the posterior circulation, intraventricular and intracerebral extension of the hematoma, and higher SBP on admission.[110] Analysis from the large International Subarachnoid Aneurysm Trial (ISAT) comparing neurosurgical clipping with endovascular coiling showed similar results.[111]

Pathophysiology

Aneurysms are more common at the bifurcation of the arteries located on the base of the brain, especially the large arteries that form the circle of Willis.[112] Hemodynamic factors that contribute to the formation and growth of aneurysms are wall shear stress

Table 4
World Federation of Neurological Surgeons grading scale

WFNS Grade	GCS	Motor Deficit
1	15	Absent
2	13 to 14	Absent
3	13 to 14	Present
4	7 to 12	Present or absent
5	3 to 6	Present or absent

Data from Report of World Federation of Neurological Surgeons committee on a universal subarachnoid hemorrhage grading scale. J Neurosurg 1988;68(6):985–6.

and hydrostatic and transmural pressures. High wall shear stress is encountered at the branch points of cerebral arteries, and long-term exposure to this could trigger vessel wall remodeling through interaction with the endothelium and the secretion of factors, such as nitric oxide and endothelial growth factors. Hydrostatic and transmural pressures produce a mechanical stretch of the wall that induces upregulation of certain molecules, such as endothelin-1B receptors, that further affect vascular smooth muscle cells by promoting apoptosis.[113] Although the mechanism of formation and growth of aneurysms is partially understood, it is still unclear what leads to aneurysmal rupture.

Clinical Presentation

The characteristic complaint of patients with SAH is a severe headache of acute onset. This headache is commonly described as "the worst headache of my life," with the highest intensity at onset. Although it is frequently accompanied by other symptoms, headache may be the only complaint in up to 40% of patients.[114] Recently, a prospective study found that the following clinical characteristics represent the highest risk of belonging to a case of SAH: age greater than 40 years, associated neck pain or stiffness, witnessed loss of consciousness, onset with exertion, vomiting, arrival by ambulance, and BP above 160/100.[115]

A subgroup of patients develops warning signs before the index SAH. The most common warning sign is again headache, which is of moderate intensity and less severe than that described in SAH. This is commonly referred to as sentinel headache or warning leak and may be associated with a small leakage of blood into the subarachnoid space or a small bleed into the aneurysmal wall. A thorough evaluation is warranted in these cases, because SAH can develop up to 110 days later.[116,117]

Physical examination may demonstrate neck stiffness and meningismus.[118] Although not specific, funduscopic evaluation may reveal subhyaloid, vitreous, or intraretinal hemorrhage (known as Terson syndrome), which is associated with higher mortality.[119] These eye findings may be found with any intracranial bleeding and are believed associated with sudden increase in ICP. Focal neurologic deficits may also be found and can be related to nerve compression by the aneurysm, intraparenchymal extension of the bleeding, or vasospasm (which typically occurs later in the course).

Diagnosis

Up to 1 in 20 SAH patients are missed during initial evaluation.[120] A high index of suspicion and a low threshold for performing diagnostic studies are key factors in making the diagnosis of SAH.

The gold standard diagnostic approach has been to initially perform a noncontrast CT scan of the brain followed by a lumbar puncture (LP) and analysis of the CSF when the CT is negative. Recently, however, some groups have suggested that current-generation multislice CT scanners as well as the availability of CTA in the acute setting may offer opportunities to selectively defer LP.[121,122]

CT

When there is clinical suspicion of SAH, the initial test of choice is a noncontrast CT scan. The sensitivity of the CT scan to detect SAH is maximal within the first 24 hours after the bleed and then decreases with time. The volume of blood in the subarachnoid space and the resolution of the scanner also influence the CT detection rate.[123] A recent multicenter prospective study of 3132 patients found that of those undergoing current-generation CT within 6 hours of symptom onset, the sensitivity was 100% (95% CI, 97%–100%) with a negative predictive value of 100% (95% CI,

99.5%–100%).[122] Noncontrast CT also provides information regarding the volume of blood, extension to the cerebral parenchyma, the presence of hydrocephalus, and the potential location of the aneurysm. Blood located in the interhemispheric fissure and the surrounding sulci has a high probability of coming from an anterior cerebral or anterior communicating artery aneurysm, whereas blood in the posterior aspect of the sylvian fissure is probably related to a middle cerebral artery aneurysm (**Fig. 3**).[123–125]

CT angiography

CTA is a fast, noninvasive, and readily available method to screen for the presence of aneurysm.[126] A recent meta-analysis showed that CTA has a pooled sensitivity of approximately 98% to detect aneurysm, with sensitivities ranging from 86% to 100%.[127] Aneurysm detection rates are related to the experience of the reviewer and aneurysmal size. Pooled specificity of CTA in this analysis reached 100% with a range of 50% to 100%.[127] Also, 3-D CTA may be as sensitive and specific as digital subtraction angiography for the detection of aneurysms (**Fig. 4**).[128] As a result, patients with negative CT/CTA have a less than 1% likelihood of aneurysmal SAH.[121] The Neurocritical Care Society recommends preferential use of CTA as an exploratory approach when it is readily available and of high technical quality over digital subtraction angiography if an immediate intervention is not planned.[129]

Lumbar puncture

LP is considered effectively 100% sensitive for detection of blood in the subarachnoid space, and it is recommended in all patients undergoing a workup for SAH with a negative CT.[130–132] CSF characteristics of SAH include an elevated opening pressure, presence of erythrocytes or red blood cells, and xanthochromia. CSF should be visually inspected for the presence of xanthochromia, a term that refers to the yellow aspect of the CSF attributable to the formation of bilirubin from the breakdown of hemoglobin in the CSF.[133]

Special consideration should be given to the use of spectrophotometry in CSF analysis for the detection of bilirubin. The use of this technique is strongly advocated in the United Kingdom, where the rate of visual assessment of the cerebrospinal fluid fell to

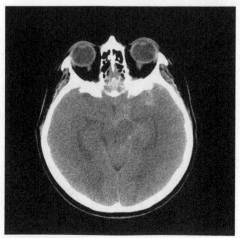

Fig. 3. SAH in the left sylvian fissure, sulci of the left hemisphere and along the left and central aspect of the suprasellar cistern, left ambient cistern, and interpenduncular cistern.

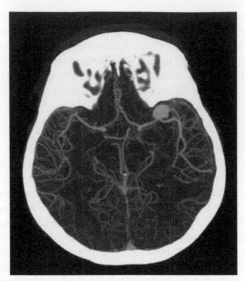

Fig. 4. 3-D reconstruction CTA on the same patient as in **Fig. 3.** An aneurysmal sac is appreciated at the distal M1 segment of the left middle cerebral artery.

6%, whereas the use of spectrophotometry rose to 94% in recent years.[134] This method has been shown to have approximately 100% sensitivity for the detection of bilirubin in patients with SAH but with low specificity.[135,136] In the United States, however, the majority of centers use visual inspection instead.[137] Some investigators recommend spectrophotometry, if available, in those cases where visual inspection yields doubtful results.[138]

Digital subtraction angiography
Digital subtraction angiography allows for direct visualization of the cerebral vasculature and remains the gold standard for detecting aneurysms. This diagnostic tool requires a dedicated neurointerventional team and provides an opportunity for therapeutic interventions as well as diagnosis.

MRI
MRI is rarely used to diagnose SAH in the ED because availability is limited, and logistical barriers to its use are much higher than with CT. Blood is not easily detectable in T1-weighted and T2-weighted MRI sequences in the acute setting, likely because the generation of deoxyhemoglobin with paramagnetic properties is delayed in the subarachnoid space.[139] The sensitivity of fluid-attenuated inversion recovery sequences, however, is comparable to that of the CT in the acute phase of an SAH and potentially superior in the subacute phase.[140,141]

Emergency Management

Airway management
The initial management of an SAH does not differ from other medical emergencies, and airway management is similar to that described previously for ICH.

Neurologic examination
During the initial evaluation, a neurologic examination should be performed and documented. Clinical grading scales that mark the severity of SAH include the Hunt and

Hess scale (**Table 5**) and the WFNS grading scale (see **Table 4**). The Hunt and Hess scale was originally designed to evaluate the operative risk of patients and to aid at deciding the best timing for neurosurgical intervention,[142] but it is now widely known and accepted as a predictor of outcome. It is based on the level of severity of clinical signs with a correlation with poor outcome with a higher grade. The WFNS grading scale uses the GCS score and groups them into 5 grades and also takes into account the presence of a motor neurologic deficit.[143]

Medical Management

Blood pressure management
When considering an optimal BP goal, an appropriate balance should be maintained. Hypotension may theoretically increase the risk of ischemia, whereas elevated BP raises the concern for aneurysmal rupture and rebleeding. Current guidelines recommend that hypotension should be avoided and that treatment of HTN should be initiated until the aneurysm is secure only with extreme BP values when the MAP is greater than 110 mm Hg, aiming at maintaining a good CPP. The recommended agents to lower BP are nicardipine, labetalol, and esmolol.[129,144]

Seizure prophylaxis
To date, no randomized controlled trial has evaluated the benefits of the prophylactic use of AEDs in patients with SAH. The incidence of seizure varies extensively in the literature.[145] Risk factors for the development of onset seizures include poor Hunt and Hess score, acute hydrocephalus, cerebral ischemia, and large volume of subarachnoid blood.[129,146,147]

Nonconvulsive seizures and nonconvulsive status epilepticus may occur after SAH, leading clinicians to recommend continuous electroencephalography monitoring in patients with poor Hunt and Hess scores.[148] Current guidelines recommend considering the use of routine AEDs, especially in patients at higher risk, and using an alternative to phenytoin, which has been linked to a poor prognosis.[129] Commonly used agents include levetiracetam, valproate, and fosphenytoin (it is unclear whether this shares the same possible negative effects as phenytoin).

Glycemic control
Both elevated and low glucose levels are associated with worse outcome after SAH. Hypoglycemia is associated with vasospasm, infarction, and more disability at 3 months. Hyperglycemia on admission and during hospitalization is also associated with poor outcome and short-term mortality.[149–151] Although a specific target glucose level has not been established, it is currently recommended to avoid hypoglycemia (serum glucose <80 mg/dL) and maintain maximum values below 200 mg/dL.[129]

Table 5 Hunt and Hess grading scale	
Grade	**Criteria**
1	Asymptomatic or minimal headache and slight nuchal rigidity
2	Moderate to severe headache, nuchalrigidity, no neurologic deficit other than cranial nerve palsy
3	Drowsiness, confusion, or mild focal neurologic deficit
4	Stupor, moderate to severe hemiparesis, possibly early decerebrate rigidity
5	Deep coma, decerebrate rigidity

Data from Hunt WE, Hess RM. Surgical risk as related to time of intervention in the repair of intracranial aneurysms. J Neurosurg 1968;28(1):14–20.

Temperature

Fever is common after SAH. Fever at admission and its presence during hospitalization are associated with poor outcome.[152] A possible infectious etiology should always be investigated, although this is uncommon during initial presentation. Medical and physical interventions can be used as therapeutic measures to reduce fever. Currently, it is recommended to initiate therapy with antipyretic agents, such as acetaminophen, when fever is present.[129] Physical surface or intravascular cooling devices should be used only when antipyretics fail, and close monitoring and treatment of shivering should be started.[129]

Vasospasm and Delayed Cerebral Ischemia

Vasospasm and delayed cerebral ischemia are deadly complications of SAH associated with poor outcome. Angiographic vasospasm occurs in up to 70% of cases.[153] Symptomatic vasospasm, associated with new focal neurologic findings and/or deterioration in the level of consciousness, occurs in approximately 30% of cases.[154] Delayed cerebral ischemia can occur days after the index SAH and can lead to neurologic deterioration and focal neurologic deficits.[155] One preventive measure is the use of oral nimodipine (60 mg by mouth or nasogastric tube every 4 hours for 21 days) and should be initiated soon after diagnosis of SAH.[156] Once vasospasm occurs, a range of medical and interventional therapies is available to maintain adequate cerebral perfusion.[129] One recognized therapy is the triple-H therapy, characterized by hypervolemia through volume expansion, HTN with BP augmentation, and hemodilution aimed at reducing blood viscosity.[157] Currently, the Neurocritical Care Society recommends that euvolemia be pursued and that the routine use of hemodilution should be reserved for cases of erythrocythemia.[129] For BP augmentation, a stepwise approach is recommended and an SBP goal of greater than 160 mm Hg or an MAP greater than 120 mm Hg is a reasonable approach.[129,158]

Aneurysm Repair

Patients with SAH require emergency neurosurgical and/or endovascular consultation. There are currently at least 2 options for the acute treatment of a ruptured aneurysm: endovascular coiling or surgical clipping. Treatment of a recently ruptured aneurysm reduces the rate of rebleeding, and the benefit is related to the time to treatment initiation.[159] Current guidelines recommend that surgical clipping or endovascular coiling should be performed to reduce the rate of rebleeding after aneurysmal SAH, and these procedures should be performed early in the disease course.[129,144]

The selection of the most appropriate intervention depends on a range of characteristics, including age, clinical status, and medical comorbidities. Aneurysm characteristics, such as location, shape, and size, are taken into consideration as well, highlighting the value of a specialized multidisciplinary group to provide care and decision making. Some expert consensus groups recommend that SAH be preferentially managed at high-volume centers (defined as those centers with greater than 60 cases of SAH per year).[129]

REFERENCES

1. van Asch CJ, Luitse MJA, Rinkel GJE, et al. Incidence, case fatality, and functional outcome of intracerebral haemorrhage over time, according to age, sex, and ethnic origin: a systematic review and meta-analysis. Lancet Neurol 2010; 9(2):167–76.

2. Aguilar MI, Freeman WD. Spontaneous intracerebral hemorrhage. Semin Neurol 2010;30(5):555–64.
3. Broderick J, Connolly S, Feldmann E, et al. Guidelines for the management of spontaneous intracerebral hemorrhage in adults. Stroke 2007;38(6):2001–23.
4. Elliott J, Smith M. The acute management of intracerebral hemorrhage: a clinical review. Anesth Analg 2010;110(5):1419–27.
5. Feigin VL, Lawes CMM, Bennett DA, et al. Worldwide stroke incidence and early case fatality reported in 56 population-based studies: a systematic review. Lancet Neurol 2009;8(4):355–69.
6. Labovitz DL, Halim A, Boden-Albala B, et al. The incidence of deep and lobar intracerebral hemorrhage in whites, blacks, and Hispanics. Neurology 2005; 65(4):518–22.
7. Ayala C, Greenlund KJ, Croft JB, et al. Racial/ethnic disparities in mortality by stroke subtype in the United States, 1995–1998. Am J Epidemiol 2001; 154(11):1057–63.
8. Qureshi AI, Giles WH, Croft JB. Racial differences in the incidence of intracerebral hemorrhage. Neurology 1999;52(8):1617.
9. Matsukawa H, Shinoda M, Fujii M, et al. Factors associated with lobar vs. nonlobar intracerebral hemorrhage. Acta Neurol Scand 2011. http://dx.doi.org/10.1111/j.1600-0404.2011.01615.x.
10. Ariesen MJ, Claus SP, Rinkel GJE, et al. Risk factors for intracerebral hemorrhage in the general population. Stroke 2003;34(8):2060–5.
11. Maia LF, Mackenzie IR, Feldman HH. Clinical phenotypes of cerebral amyloid angiopathy. J Neurol Sci 2007;257(1–2):23–30.
12. Badjatia N, Rosand J. Intracerebral hemorrhage. Neurologist 2005;11(6): 311–24.
13. Wieberdink RG, Poels MMF, Vernooij MW, et al. Serum lipid levels and the risk of intracerebral hemorrhage: the Rotterdam Study. Arterioscler Thromb Vasc Biol 2011;31(12):2982–9.
14. Biffi A, Sonni A, Anderson CD, et al. Variants at APOE influence risk of deep and lobar intracerebral hemorrhage. Ann Neurol 2010;68(6):934–43.
15. Brouwers HB, Biffi A, Ayres AM, et al. Apolipoprotein e genotype predicts hematoma expansion in lobar intracerebral hemorrhage. Stroke 2012;43(6):1490–5.
16. Flaherty ML. Anticoagulant-associated intracerebral hemorrhage. Semin Neurol 2010;30(5):565–72.
17. Martin-Schild S, Albright KC, Hallevi H, et al. Intracerebral hemorrhage in cocaine users. Stroke 2010;41(4):680–4.
18. Fisher CM. Pathological observations in hypertensive cerebral hemorrhage. J Neuropathol Exp Neurol 1971;30(3):536–50.
19. Vinters H. Cerebral amyloid angiopathy. A critical review. Stroke 1987;18(2): 311–24.
20. Viswanathan A, Greenberg SM. Cerebral amyloid angiopathy in the elderly. Ann Neurol 2011;70(6):871–80.
21. Aronowski J, Zhao X. Molecular pathophysiology of cerebral hemorrhage: secondary brain injury. Stroke 2011;42(6):1781–6.
22. Brott T, Broderick J, Kothari R, et al. Early hemorrhage growth in patients with intracerebral hemorrhage. Stroke 1997;28(1):1–5.
23. Runchey S, Mc Gee S. Clinical findings distinguishing hemorrhagic stroke from ischemic stroke. JAMA 2010;30(22):2280–6.
24. Panagos PD, Jauch EC, Broderick JP. Intracerebral hemorrhage. Emerg Med Clin North Am 2002;20(3):631–55.

The job of the emergency physician is difficult. The first area of difficulty begins with the type of emergency department (ED) and the availability of resources that the emergency physician has at his/her disposal. Academic EDs that are designated as stroke centers have a stroke team that is activated by the emergency physician. A stroke neurologist is immediately available to assess the patient and a radiologist to interpret the computed tomography (CT) of the head. The stroke neurologist decides on further imaging (CT angiogram or magnetic resonance imaging [MRI]), thrombolysis, or interventional therapy. Academic centers have 24-hour availability of CT angiograms and/or MRI. Interventional capability through either a neurointerventional physician or an interventional radiologist is also available. Alternatively, community and rural hospitals may have only 1 emergency physician working, with or without a neurologist available for telephone consultation. In some rural EDs, night staffing is with physician extenders or physicians who are not trained in EM. Radiology services for interpreting CT studies may be outsourced to radiologists elsewhere in the United States or even abroad. The emergency physician or physician extender in these circumstances must be able to review CT studies and decide on initiating thrombolysis with rtPA. The emergency provider in this setting then has a far more complex role in determining if a stroke mimic exists.

The actual number of patients who present with a stroke mimic compared with those with true stroke varies depending on the research study that deals with this question. A prospectively collected stroke/MRI data bank in Germany from 2004 to 2010, had 42 of 648 (6.5%) patients suspected with ischemic stroketreated with rtPA with a final diagnosis of a stroke mimic.[4] Stroke mimic diagnoses included 20 patients with seizures, 7 patients with conversion disorders, 6 patients with dementia, 3 patients with migraine headache, 2 patients with brain tumors, and 4 other cases.[4] Complications from rtPA therapy occurred in only 1 of the patients in this study (orolingual edema).[4] Chernyshev and colleagues[5] found that 14% of the treated patients were eventually diagnosed with a stroke mimic and none suffered a complication from thrombolytic therapy. This group of patients only included those treated in the 3-hour window from symptom onset.

Little attention has been paid to patients presenting with transient ischemic attacks (TIAs) and conditions mimicking TIA. In a single center, prospective cohort study over 2 years in Switzerland, approximately 20% of patients suspected with TIA at presentation were TIA mimics.[6] This article does not discuss about TIA mimics.

This article describes the common stroke mimic presentations by cause, including toxic-metabolic pathologies, seizure disorders, degenerative neurologic conditions, and peripheral neuropathies. These conditions are not immediately obvious to the treating physician, and he/she has to rely on history taking, laboratory analysis, and neuroimaging studies to elucidate possible stroke mimics. Even with a stroke team comprising a neurologist and neuroradiologist assisting the emergency physician, patients with stroke mimics will not always be immediately identified.

TOXIC-METABOLIC

Glycemic imbalance can present in the form of high or low blood glucose level.

Hypoglycemia can be loosely defined as low blood glucose levels with changes in the mental status. The most commonly cited laboratory values for hypoglycemia in diabetics is a blood glucose level of less than 70 mg/dL, with presence of signs or symptoms consistent with low blood glucose level, as well as the resolution of symptoms with the correction of low blood glucose level.[7] Although the correction of hypoglycemia should be accompanied by the resolution of symptoms, neurologic symptoms may linger somewhat after glucose treatment.[8] In healthy individuals, a level of less than 55 mg/dL of blood glucose has been used as the threshold for hypoglycemia although it can present at lower levels if there have been previous recurrent episodes of hypoglycemia.[9] Patients may exhibit signs and symptoms that may be confused with a cerebrovascular accident when truly presenting with isolated hypoglycemia.[10] As blood glucose level becomes dangerously low, patients may present with confusion, altered behavioral patterns, seizure, and/or coma. Foster and Hart[11] exemplify the focal neurologic deficit in the setting of hypoglycemia with a study of 2 patients with recurrent presentations of hemiplegia. On each presentation, symptoms were corrected with a reduction in insulin dosing and workups including angiography were negative for a primary neurologic event.[11] One study showed a 2% prevalence of hypoglycemic hemiparesis although there was concomitant evidence of vascular disease in these patients.[3] In subsequent reviews, hypoglycemic hemiplegia has been unreliably associated with vascular disease.[4] Right-sided hemiparesis is more common than left sided, and right-sided hemiparesis often has associated aphasia.[4]

Hyperglycemia is also capable of producing focal neurologic deficits. Many patients regularly have an elevated level of blood glucose, but neurologic changes may occur when it becomes pathologic, such as in diabetic ketoacidosis or hyperosmolar hyperglycemic nonketotic state. This condition is more common in patients with nonketotic hyperglycemia in whom metabolic encephalopathy can develop, with involvement of the cortex, brain stem, and spinal cord leading to neurologic signs.[4] Maccario[12] thought focal deficits, including homonymous hemianopsia, hemiplegia, hemisensory deficits, and aphasia, were caused by cellular hyperosmolarity.

Metabolic imbalances, such as hypernatremia,[5] hyponatremia, and hepatic encephalopathy, may also cause focal neurologic deficits.[5,6] Hypernatremia is similar to hyperglycemia in its effect of cerebral hyperosmolarity and the resultant encephalopathy due to failure of thirst, antidiuretic hormone secretion, and initially slow onset of corrective idiogenic osmoles to abate cellular shrinkage.[4,5] Hyponatremia causes encephalopathy through cellular swelling, but can be acute or insidious in onset, with acute onset more often associated with neurologic changes. Hepatic encephalopathy has been rarely documented as causing focal neurologic deficits, but in a study by Cadranel and colleagues,[13] 17.4% of patients with hepatic encephalopathy over a 12-month period showed neurologic deficits. This included 48 episodes of encephalopathy due to liver pathology with 8 instances of resolved focal neurologic deficits with the resolution of hepatic encephalopathy. Patients were most commonly found to have hemiparesis and hemiplegia, noted in comatose patients because of decreased movement with painful stimuli. All patients with documented neurologic signs had negative head CT and lumbar puncture, but not all had brain MRI and/or echo Doppler studies of the neck. There was no prognostic significance of patients who did show neurologic deficits versus those who did not in the outcome of the hepatic encephalopathy. These neurologic deficits had not previously been well noted in the literature, but the investigators thought it was important for physicians to be aware of this presentation.[13]

INGESTIONS

Patients presenting with altered mental status and an atypical neurologic examination should raise suspicion for ingestion, including use of illicit drugs, misuse of prescription medications, overdose of any medication, or drug interactions. Toxicologic screening including, but not limited to, salicylates and acetaminophen, as well as opiates or other illicit drugs capable of sedation or unusual behaviors is essential. An electrocardiogram is essential to assess for cardiac dysrhythmias caused by medications and to check the PR interval and QTc interval for concerning cardiac results of ingestion. Ingestions are a diagnosis of exclusion in the acutely altered patient and should be ruled out while working up the possibility of a true neurologic event.

SEIZURE AND TODD PARALYSIS

Along with hypoglycemia, seizure has been noted as the most common presenting condition resulting in a stroke mimic.[8,9] Patients with focal seizures, even if progressing to generalized seizures, can present with hemiparesis, often referred to as Todd paresis; gaze deviation; and decreased mental status. The cause of Todd paresis is attributed to increased metabolic demand from the active depletion of the excitatory neurons in the postictal state.[10] Rupprecht and colleagues[14] studied postictal dysfunction using cranial perfusion MRI scans and found evidence of early global hemispheric perfusion mismatch without lasting injury. MRI at 10 hours show full resolution, with interval hyperperfusion. Changes are not associated with a particular vascular distribution but rather associated with the epileptic focus and surrounding tissue.[11,12]

MIGRAINE HEADACHE

Migraine headache is a recurrent throbbing headache, either unilateral or bilateral, that can have a prolonged course with associated visual and auditory irritation, and up to 25% of patients with migraine exhibit focal neurologic deficits.[15–17] Migraine has a similar causative function as seizures in the focal neurologic deficit masking as a stroke.[13,16] The pathophysiology is termed cortical spreading depression, with the excitation of neurons and subsequent inhibition.[13,16,18] One subtype of migraine is the hemiplegic migraine, which can be either sporadic or genetically inherited and is defined by an aura accompanied by motor weakness. They often progress throughout a patient's lifetime with the gradual worsening of visual, sensory, aphasia, and cerebellar symptoms. Patients diagnosed with hemiplegic migraines may experience headache without these neurologic deficits. Most aspects of the hemiplegic migraine are self-resolving, but in a small number of patients, it causes permanent neurologic changes.[18]

DEGENERATIVE NEUROLOGIC DISORDERS, MULTIPLE SCLEROSIS, OPTIC NEURITIS

Degenerative neurologic disorders occur in many forms, including multiple sclerosis (MS) and leukoencephalopathy from viruses, medications, or ingestions. The resultant demyelination from these disorders can present with hemiparesis, cranial nerve palsies, and vision disturbances. The most discussed demyelinating disease is MS, in which a small subset of patients suffers from brief paroxysmal symptoms, such as dysarthria, ataxia, diplopia, and sensory deficits, which are a less common feature of disseminated sclerosis.[14,19–21] Researchers have found the responsible lesions at the level of the midbrain or below, as shown on MRI scans of patients in the paroxysmal dysarthria-ataxia subgroups.[20,22] These attacks are usually well controlled and have a dramatic improvement with carbamazepine.[14,20,22,23]

A well-described postinfectious or postimmunization cause of demyelination is acute demyelination encephalomyelitis (ADEM),[24] which is more common in children, and an immune-mediated process. Differentiation between ADEM and MS has been studied more commonly in children, but ADEM is noted to have a shorter onset of about 5 days and is monophasic compared with approximately 2 weeks with MS and is chronic.[24,25] Demyelination has also been noted in patients with JC virus, which has been associated with progressive multifocal leukoencephalopathy, in immunocompromised hosts. Most individuals are carriers by adulthood, up to 80%, but JC virus focus its attack in patients with CD8 + deficiency.[26,27]

Optic neuritis, which is a demyelinating condition of the optic nerve, may be present bilaterally, but is more commonly unilateral in MS and bilateral in ADEM.[25] Bilateral presentation is also more common in children compared with adults with acute demyelinating optic neuritis.[28] In MS, 15% to 20% of patients initially present with optic neuritis and about 50% of all patients with MS develop optic neuritis at some time.[28,29] Presentation is often subacute, with loss of red-vision in particular, visual field loss and an afferent papillary defect are often present as well.[28]

Myelopathy is a pathologic condition that affects the spinal cord, leading to motor or sensory loss. Acute myelopathy is defined as having maximum effect within 4 weeks of onset. Causative factors include trauma, compressive lesions, vascular lesions, infection or inflammation, and toxic, paraneoplastic, or electrical injuries.[30] Acute myelopathies are often diagnosed when the patient does not have the hallmark findings of MS, including the typical MRI findings of demyelinating lesions, leading to a broader differential diagnosis. Inflammatory changes of the spinal cord are most commonly due to direct or postinfectious causes and other autoimmune demyelinating diseases, such as ADEM.[31–33] Inflammatory myelitis can cause acute transverse myelitis, and likely causes include viral, bacterial, postvaccination, and autoimmune diseases; MS; paraneoplastic syndromes; or idiopathic. Bacterial pathogens such as mycoplasma, tuberculosis, Lyme, and syphilis may also lead to myelitis.[33,34] *Treponema pallidum* was the most common cause before the discovery of antibiotics.[35] Symptoms of transverse myelitis include weakness in the legs, increase in pain sensation (allodynia), changes in bowel or bladder control, and, less commonly, sensory changes.[32] Infectious myelopathies are less common, with HIV being the most common cause of infectious myelopathies. Viral causes include herpes simplex and zoster, enteroviruses, human T-cell lymphotropic virus type I, and mycobacterium.

CEREBROVASCULAR NARROWING

The primary causes of cerebrovascular narrowing include central nervous system (CNS) vasculitis, reversible cerebral vasoconstriction syndrome, aneurysmal subarachnoid hemorrhage, and atherosclerosis. Primary CNS vasculitis and reversible cerebral vasoconstriction have similar angiographic findings but are separate entities with differing implications.[36] Vasculitis of the CNS is a rare and poorly understood entity, which was first described in 1959 by Cravioto and Feigin.[37] Since that time, only about 500 cases have been identified.[38] Diagnosis of primary angiitis of the CNS (PACNS) is increasing because of more recent awareness and improved imaging technology, but the case numbers remain small. PACNS is most commonly found in men in the fifth decade of life.[38] Onset of PACNS is variable from acute to chronic and, in some cases, may mimic chronic meningitis. PACNS is usually a multivessel disease affecting varied cerebral territories. Signs and symptoms range from visual changes secondary to cranial nerve involvement to ataxia and myelopathies, often in conjunction with constitutional systemic manifestations. It is estimated that 30% to 50% of patients diagnosed with PACNS ultimately have TIAs and strokes secondary to the *vascular changes*.[38–40]

Reversible cerebral vasoconstriction syndrome (RCVS) is characterized by a thunderclap headache and may or may not be associated with neurologic findings. Young women between the ages of 20and 50 are most commonly affected and frequently have a past medical history of migraine headaches.[41] There is a small, but significant, morbidity associated with RCVS that may result in ischemic or hemorrhagic stroke. Although a stroke may result from vasoconstriction, this condition being reversible, by its definition, often leaves most patients with few long-term adverse outcomes.[36] There are several subsets of syndromes in RCVS, but the essential finding is vaso-spasm of the cerebral vessels, resolving over days to weeks. Inciting factors include trauma, hypertension, sympathomimetic drugs, and cerebral tumors. Marijuana, cocaine, nicotine patches, selective serotonin reuptake inhibitors, and nasal decon-gestants, such as pseudoephedrine and ephedrine, are all associated with RCVS. Neurologic effects from vasoconstriction can vary and involve the brain territory supplied by the constricted artery, causing signs and symptoms, such as dysarthria, hemiplegia, hemisensory deficits, aphasia, visual changes, and more.[39,42] Hemor-rhagic or ischemic stroke has been cited with persistent vasoconstriction and is the major determinant of morbidity and mortality in these patients.[36,42]

Idiopathic intracranial hypertension (IIH), previously known as pseudotumor cerebri, is a syndrome that often afflicts young, obese women,[43,44] and is characterized by increased intracranial pressures in the absence of structural cerebral changes including obstruction, mass, vascular lesions or changes in the cerebrospinal fluid (CSF).[45] IIH was initially a "benign" condition, but Corbett and Thompson[58] demon-strated the destructive vision changes caused by papilledema, which lead to a change in the nomenclature from benign intracranial hypertension to IIH. Decreased vision stems from optic atrophy as a direct result of increased intracranial pressure. Approx-imately 25% of patients with IIH experience such vision disturbances.[47] Patients with IIH most commonly present with headache and often experience visual obscurations and less commonly double vision and blurry vision.[44,47] Approximately 35%to 70% of patients experience visual symptoms.[44,48,49] Abducens nerve is the most commonly affected cranial nerve[44] and was previously included in the presenting signs of IIH according to the Modified Dandy Criteria.[50] The criteria has since been updated by Friedman and Jacobson[51] and VI nerve palsy is no longer explicitly included in the definition[45] but is nonetheless still often present. Occurring in about 80% of cases, IV nerve palsy is caused by increased pressure on the nerve from increased intracra-nial pressure, causing mass effect.[52] Facial nerve,[51,53–55] oculomotor,[56,57] troch-lear,[46,58] and trigeminal nerve palsies[57,59] have all been observed infrequently in patients with IIH.[60] Papilledema is present in most patients, but its absence does not exclude the diagnosis of IIH.[52,61–71]

PERIPHERAL NEUROPATHIES

Peripheral neuropathies are due to cellular changes in nerves that lie outside the brain, spinal cord, and CNS. These include small to large diameter nerves innervating either motor or sensory systems. Because of their anatomic distribution and placement in proximity to bony foramina and ligamentous spaces, they are susceptible not only to ischemic, toxic or autoimmune damage, but also to bony compression and entrap-ment. Three main types of degeneration exist including axonal degeneration, seg-mental degeneration, and wallerian degeneration. Axonal degenerationdamages the myelin distally and the axis cylinder. Segmental degeneration has myelin damage but axonal sparing. Wallerian degeneration is from a direct injury to the nerve resulting in distal degeneration due to the separation from the cell body. Main symp-toms include motor dysfunction, muscle atrophy, loss of sensation and reflexes, paresthesias, and pain. Neuropathies include mononeuropathies, polyneuropathies, radiculopathies, and plexopathies, which involve multiple nerves within a plexus. The vast networks of peripheral neurons mean there is a multitude of neural pathologic condition. These can be differentiated from the pathologic conditions of the CNS through physical examination, radiological imaging of the brain, electromyography, nerve biopsy, and CSF and blood testing. Often, this extent of testing requires more time than an initial emergency department visit to make such a diagnosis with certainty. Guillain-Barre Syndrome is an ascending paralysis that is divided into several subtypes characterized by symmetric peripheral weakness, areflexia, increased protein levels in the CSF and a progressive ascending course of motor weakness.

SUMMARY

Stroke mimics are an important consideration for emergency physicians and physician extenders working in EDs. Even with a time window of 4.5 hours, the work-up must often be accelerated depending on the time at which the patient presents to the ED. As previously noted, the resources available to emergency providers differ greatly across the country. Nevertheless, it is incumbent on the emergency provider to think stroke first and proceed accordingly.

REFERENCES

1. Roger VL, Go AS, Lloyd-Jones DM, et al. Heart disease and stroke statistics–2011 update: a report from the American Heart Association. Circulation 2011; 123(4):e18–209.
2. Goldstein LB, Bushnell CD, Adams RJ, et al. Guidelines for the primary prevention of stroke: a guideline for healthcare professionals from the American Heart Association/American Stroke Association. Stroke 2010;42:517–84.
3. Hacke W, Kaste M, Bluhmki E, et al. Thrombolysis with alteplase 3 to 4.5 hours after acute ischemic stroke. N Engl J Med 2008;359:1317–29.
4. Forster A, Griebe M, Wolf ME, et al. How to identify stroke mimics in patients eligible for intravenous thrombolysis? J Neurol 2012 [Epub ahead of print]. http://www.ncbi.nlm.nih.gov/pubmed/22231865. Accessed April 14, 2012.
5. Chernyshev OY, Martin-Schild S, Albright KC, et al. Safety of tPA in stroke mimics and neuroimaging-negative cerebral ischemia. Neurology 2010;74(17):1340–5.
6. Amort M, Fluri F, Schafer J, et al. Transient ischemic attack versus transient ischemic attack mimics: frequency, clinical characteristics, and outcome. Cerebrovasc Dis 2011;32(1):57–64 [Epub 2011 May 25].
7. Cryer PE, Axelrod L, Grossman AB, et al. Evaluation and management of adult hypoglycemic disorders: an endocrine society clinical practice guideline. J Clin Endocrinol Metab 2009;94(3):709–28. http://dx.doi.org/10.1210/jc.2008-1410.
8. Cryer PE. Hypoglycemia, functional brain failure, and brain death. J Clin Invest 2007;117(4):868–70. http://dx.doi.org/10.1172/JCI31669.
9. Cryer PE. The prevention and correction of hypoglycemia. In: Jefferson LS, Cherrington A, Goodman HM, editors. Handbook of physiology; section 7, the endocrine system. volume II. The endocrine pancreas and regulation of metabolism. New York: Oxford University Press; 2001. p. 1057–92.
10. Malouf R, Brust JC. Hypoglycemia: causes, neurological manifestations, and outcome. Ann Neurol 1985;17(5):421–30. http://dx.doi.org/10.1002/ana.410170502.
11. Foster JW, Hart RG. Hypoglycemic hemiplegia: two cases and a clinical review. Stroke 1987;18(5):944–6.

12. Maccario M. Neurological dysfunction associated with nonketotic hyperglycemia. Arch Neurol 1968;19(5):525–34.

13. Cadranel JF, Lebiez E, Di Martino V, et al. Focal neurological signs in hepatic encephalopathy in cirrhotic patients: an underestimated entity? Am J Gastroenterol 2001;96(2):515–8. http://dx.doi.org/10.1111/j.1572-0241.2001.03552.x.

14. Rupprecht S, Schwab M, Fitzek C, et al. Hemispheric hypoperfusion in postictal paresis mimics early brain ischemia. Epilepsy Res 2010;89(2-3):355–9. http://dx.doi.org/10.1016/j.eplepsyres.2010.02.009.

15. Guisado R, Arieff AI. Neurologic manifestations of diabetic comas: correlation with biochemical alterations in the brain. Metabolism 1975;24(5):665–79.

16. Samuels MA, Seifter JL. Encephalopathies caused by electrolyte disorders. Semin Neurol 2011;31(2):135–8. http://dx.doi.org/10.1055/s-0031-1277983.

17. Libman RB, Wirkowski E, Alvir J, et al. Conditions that mimic stroke in the emergency department. Implications for acute stroke trials. Arch Neurol 1995;52(11):1119–22.

18. Goldstein LB, Simel DL. Is this patient having a stroke? JAMA 2005;293(19): 2391–402. http://dx.doi.org/10.1001/jama.293.19.2391.

19. Norris JW, Hachinski VC. Misdiagnosis of stroke. Lancet 1982;1(8267):328–31.

20. Todd RB. The lumleian lectures for 1849. On the pathology and treatment of convulsive diseases. Epilepsia 2005;46(7):995–1009. http://dx.doi.org/10.1111/j.1528-1167.2005.10205.x.

21. Leonhardt G, de Greiff A, Weber J, et al. Brain perfusion following single seizures. Epilepsia 2005;46(12):1943–9. http://dx.doi.org/10.1111/j.1528-1167.2005.00336.x.

22. Cutrer F. New information in our evolving understanding of migraine aura and cortical spreading depression. Cephalalgia 2009;29(10):1129–31. http://dx.doi.org/10.1111/j.1468-2982.2009.01985.x.

23. Cutrer FM. Pathophysiology of migraine. Semin Neurol 2010;30(2):120–30. http://dx.doi.org/10.1055/s-0030-1249222.

24. Headache Classification Subcommittee of the International Headache Society. The international classification of headache disorders: 2nd edition. Cephalalgia 2004;24(Suppl 1):9–160.

25. Smith JM, Bradley DP, James MF, et al. Physiological studies of cortical spreading depression. Biol Rev Camb Philos Soc 2006;81(4):457–81. http://dx.doi.org/10.1017/S1464793106007081.

26. Russell MB, Ducros A. Sporadic and familial hemiplegic migraine: pathophysiological mechanisms, clinical characteristics, diagnosis, and management. Lancet Neurol 2011;10(5):457–70. http://dx.doi.org/10.1016/S1474-4422(11)70048-5.

27. Espir ML, Watkins SM, Smith HV. Paroxysmal dysarthria and other transient neurological disturbances in disseminated sclerosis. J Neurol Neurosurg Psychiatry 1966;29(4):323–30.

28. Marcel C, Anheim M, Flamand-Rouviere C, et al. Symptomatic paroxysmal dysarthria-ataxia in demyelinating diseases. J Neurol 2010;257(8):1369–72. http://dx.doi.org/10.1007/s00415-010-5534-3.

29. Twomey JA, Espir ML. Paroxysmal symptoms as the first manifestations of multiple sclerosis. J Neurol Neurosurg Psychiatry 1980;43(4):296–304.

30. Ostermann PO, Westerberg CE. Paroxysmal attacks in multiple sclerosis. Brain 1975;98(2):189–202.

31. Li Y, Zeng C, Luo T. Paroxysmal dysarthria and ataxia in multiple sclerosis and corresponding magnetic resonance imaging findings. J Neurol 2011;258(2): 273–6. http://dx.doi.org/10.1007/s00415-010-5748-4.

32. Matthews WB. Paroxysmal symptoms in multiple sclerosis. J Neurol Neurosurg Psychiatry 1975;38(6):617–23.
33. Tenembaum S, Chitnis T, Ness J, et al, International Pediatric MS Study Group. Acute disseminated encephalomyelitis. Neurology 2007;68(16 Suppl 2):S23–36. http://dx.doi.org/10.1212/01.wnl.0000259404.51352.7f.
34. Palace J. Acute disseminated encephalomyelitis and its place amongst other acute inflammatory demyelinating CNS disorders. J Neurol Sci 2011;306(1–2):188–91. http://dx.doi.org/10.1016/j.jns.2011.03.028.
35. Du Pasquier RA, Kuroda MJ, Zheng Y, et al. A prospective study demonstrates an association between JC virus-specific cytotoxic T lymphocytes and the early control of progressive multifocal leukoencephalopathy. Brain 2004;127(Pt 9):1970–8. http://dx.doi.org/10.1093/brain/awh215.
36. Tyler KL. Emerging viral infections of the central nervous system: Part 2. Arch Neurol 2009;66(9):1065–74. http://dx.doi.org/10.1001/archneurol.2009.189.
37. Cravioto H, Feigin I. Noninfectious granulomatous angiitis with a predilection for the nervous system. Neurology 1959;9:599–609.
38. Arnold AC. Evolving management of optic neuritis and multiple sclerosis. Am J Ophthalmol 2005;139(6):1101–8. http://dx.doi.org/10.1016/j.ajo.2005.01.031.
39. Ghezzi A, Baldini SM, Zaffaroni M. Differential diagnosis of acute myelopathies. Neurol Sci 2001;22(Suppl 2):S60–4.
40. Frohman EM, Wingerchuk DM. Clinical practice. Transverse myelitis. N Engl J Med 2010;363(6):564–72. http://dx.doi.org/10.1056/NEJMcp1001112.
41. Kaplin AI, Krishnan C, Deshpande DM, et al. Diagnosis and management of acute myelopathies. Neurologist 2005;11(1):2–18. http://dx.doi.org/10.1097/01.nrl.0000149975.39201.0b.
42. Andersen O. Myelitis. Curr Opin Neurol 2000;13(3):311–6.
43. Jeffery DR, Mandler RN, Davis LE. Transverse myelitis. Retrospective analysis of 33 cases, with differentiation of cases associated with multiple sclerosis and parainfectious events. Arch Neurol 1993;50(5):532–5.
44. Berger JR, Sabet A. Infectious myelopathies. Semin Neurol 2002;22(2):133–42. http://dx.doi.org/10.1055/s-2002-36536.
45. Calabrese LH, Dodick DW, Schwedt TJ, et al. Narrative review: reversible cerebral vasoconstriction syndromes. Ann Intern Med 2007;146(1):34–44.
46. Corbett JJ, Savino PJ, Thompson HS, et al. Visual loss in pseudotumor cerebri. Follow-up of 57 patients from five to 41 years and a profile of 14 patients with permanent severe visual loss. Arch Neurol 1982;39(8):461–74.
47. Hajj-Ali RA, Singhal AB, Benseler S, et al. Primary angiitis of the CNS. Lancet Neurol 2011;10(6):561–72. http://dx.doi.org/10.1016/S1474-4422(11)70081-3.
48. Calabrese LH, Duna GF, Lie JT. Vasculitis in the central nervous system. Arthritis Rheum 1997;40(7):1189–201.
49. Salvarani C, Brown RD Jr, Calamia KT, et al. Primary central nervous system vasculitis: analysis of 101 patients. Ann Neurol 2007;62(5):442–51. http://dx.doi.org/10.1002/ana.21226.
50. Singhal AB. Cerebral vasoconstriction syndromes. Top Stroke Rehabil 2004;11(2):1–6.
51. Friedman DI, Jacobson DM. Diagnostic criteria for idiopathic intracranial hypertension. Neurology 2002;59(10):1492–5.
52. Sattar A, Manousakis G, Jensen MB. Systematic review of reversible cerebral vasoconstriction syndrome. Expert Rev Cardiovasc Ther 2010;8(10):1417–21. http://dx.doi.org/10.1586/erc.10.124.

53. Durcan FJ, Corbett JJ, Wall M. The incidence of pseudotumor cerebri. Population studies in Iowa and louisiana. Arch Neurol 1988;45(8):875–7.
54. Wall M, George D. Idiopathic intracranial hypertension. A prospective study of 50 patients. Brain 1991;114(Pt 1A):155–80.
55. Corbett JJ, Thompson HS. The rational management of idiopathic intracranial hypertension. Arch Neurol 1989;46(10):1049–51.
56. Dhungana S, Sharrack B, Woodroofe N. Idiopathic intracranial hypertension. Acta Neurol Scand 2010;121(2):71–82. http://dx.doi.org/10.1111/j.1600-0404.2009. 01172.x.
57. Weisberg LA. Benign intracranial hypertension. Medicine (Baltimore) 1975;54(3): 197–207.
58. Smith JL. Whence pseudotumor cerebri? J Clin Neuroophthalmol 1985;5(1):55–6.
59. Binder DK, Horton JC, Lawton MT, et al. Idiopathic intracranial hypertension. Neurosurgery 2004;54(3):538–51 [discussion: 551–2].
60. Chutorian AM, Gold AP, Braun CW. Benign intracranial hypertension and bell's palsy. N Engl J Med 1977;296(21):1214–5. http://dx.doi.org/10.1056/ NEJM197705262962107.
61. Davie C, Kennedy P, Katifi HA. Seventh nerve palsy as a false localising sign. J Neurol Neurosurg Psychiatry 1992;55(6):510–1.
62. Kiwak KJ, Levine SE. Benign intracranial hypertension and facial diplegia. Arch Neurol 1984;41(7):787–8.
63. Snyder DA, Frenkel M. An unusual presentation of pseudotumor cerebri. Ann Ophthalmol 1979;11(12):1823–7.
64. McCammon A, Kaufman HH, Sears ES. Transient oculomotor paralysis in pseudotumor cerebri. Neurology 1981;31(2):182–4.
65. Chari C, Rao NS. Benign intracranial hypertension–its unusual manifestations. Headache 1991;31(9):599–600.
66. Halpern JI, Gordon WH Jr. Trochlear nerve palsy as a false localizing sign. Ann Ophthalmol 1981;13(1):53–6.
67. Lee AG. Fourth nerve palsy in pseudotumor cerebri. Strabismus 1995;3(2):57–9. http://dx.doi.org/10.3109/09273979509063835.
68. Davenport RJ, Will RG, Galloway PJ. Isolated intracranial hypertension presenting with trigeminal neuropathy. J Neurol Neurosurg Psychiatry 1994;57(3):381.
69. Capobianco DJ, Brazis PW, Cheshire WP. Idiopathic intracranial hypertension and seventh nerve palsy. Headache 1997;37(5):286–8.
70. Krishna R, Kosmorsky GS, Wright KW. Pseudotumor cerebri sine papilledema with unilateral sixth nerve palsy. J Neuroophthalmol 1998;18(1):53–5.
71. Lipton HL, Michelson PE. Pseudotumor cerebri syndrome without papilledema. JAMA 1972;220(12):1591–2.

Pediatric Stroke

Charise L. Freundlich, MD[a], Anna M. Cervantes-Arslanian, MD[b],
David H. Dorfman, MD[a],*

KEYWORDS

- Pediatric stroke • Thrombolytic therapy • Risk factors • Arterial ischemic stroke

KEY POINTS

- Stroke is rare in children but leads to significant morbidity and mortality.
- Emergency department physicians are likely to be the first to evaluate children suffering from a stroke and it is, therefore, important for them to recognize common presenting features and risk factors for pediatric stroke.
- Further research is needed on the acute and preventative treatments of pediatric stroke because merely applying our knowledge of stroke in adults to children is insufficient.

INTRODUCTION

Stroke is uncommon in the pediatric population. Children from neonates to adolescents may suffer from strokes, with the stroke type varying according to age. Certain children with underlying disorders are at a particular risk. Furthermore, stroke may present differently in children compared with adults. The World Health Organization defines stroke as a clinical syndrome of rapidly developing focal or global disturbance in brain function lasting more than 24 hours or leading to brain tissue death with no obvious nonvascular cause.[1] This definition excludes much of what defines stroke in children. In children, brain infarction may occur on imaging despite only transient symptoms; antecedent or ongoing infection may be associated with stroke; and in cerebral venous sinus thrombosis, isolated headache without focal neurologic disturbance may occur.[1]

Emergency department (ED) physicians are likely to be the first physicians to evaluate these patients and it is, therefore, important for them to recognize common presenting features and risk factors for pediatric stroke. The following review is intended to describe the epidemiology, clinical presentations, stroke types, associated risk

[a] Division of Pediatric Emergency Medicine, Boston University School of Medicine/Boston Medical Center, 72 East Concord Street, Boston, MA 02118, USA; [b] Department of Neurology, Boston University School of Medicine/Boston Medical Center, 72 East Concord Street, Boston, MA 02118, USA
* Corresponding author.
E-mail address: david.dorfman@bmc.org

Emerg Med Clin N Am 30 (2012) 805–828
doi:10.1016/j.emc.2012.05.005
0733-8627/12/$ – see front matter © 2012 Elsevier Inc. All rights reserved.

factors, evaluation, treatment, and prognosis of pediatric stroke. A review of the literature on the use of thrombolytics in children and other therapies for stroke in children are discussed.

EPIDEMIOLOGY OF PEDIATRIC STROKE

A recent estimate of the incidence of pediatric stroke is 2 to 13 per 100,000 children per year.[1] Agrawal and colleagues[2] used a retrospective search strategy of radiology studies in addition to a search based on diagnostic coding for stroke to look at a population of 2.3 million children aged younger than 20 years in Northern California from 1993 to 2003 and found that the incidence of arterial ischemic stroke was 2.4 per 100,000 children per year, which is significantly higher than prior estimates.[2] Hemorrhagic stroke accounts for approximately half of all childhood stroke, whereas childhood cerebral venous sinus thrombosis (CVST) is rare, with an incidence of 0.67 per 100,000 children per year.[1] Gender and ethnic disparities are noted in several studies, with boys and black children at a higher risk for stroke than girls and other ethnic groups.[3,4]

PEDIATRIC ARTERIAL ISCHEMIC STROKE

Significant prehospital and in-hospital delays often exist in diagnosing children with stroke, stressing the need for educating ED physicians about pediatric stroke. In a study of 209 children aged 1 month to 18 years with arterial ischemic stroke (AIS) at the Hospital for Sick Children in Toronto, the median interval from symptom onset to AIS diagnosis was 22.7 hours. Prehospital delay (symptom onset to hospital arrival) was 1.7 hours, whereas the in-hospital delay (presentation to diagnosis) was 12.7 hours. The diagnosis of AIS was suspected on the initial assessment in only 38% of these children and only 20% were diagnosed within 6 hours. Obstacles to timely diagnosis included the lack of experience with pediatric stroke in the ED, frequent nonfocal presentations of stroke in children, a wider differential diagnosis for focal neurologic deficits in childhood, and the poor sensitivity of acute computed tomography scanning for the diagnosis of pediatric AIS.[5]

AIS in Infants and Older Children

Presentation
Children aged less than 1 year with AIS may present with focal weakness but are more likely than older children to present with seizures and altered mental status. As in adults, older children usually have hemiparesis or other focal neurologic signs, such as aphasia, visual disturbance, or cerebellar signs. Speech abnormalities and headache are difficult to detect in children aged less than 1 year because of minimal or absent expressive speech ability in this age group.[6]

Cause
Approximately half of the children presenting with AIS have at least one identifiable predisposing cause. The International Pediatric Stroke Study (IPSS) prospectively enrolled 676 children aged 29 days to 18 years with AIS. In 9% of the children, no identifiable risk factor was present. The most frequent risk factors included arteriopathies (53%), cardiac disorders (31%), and infection (24%). Other common risk factors include blood disorders and genetic conditions.[7]

In other studies, up to 30% of children with AIS have no known risk factor. The most common underlying conditions are sickle cell disease (SCD) arteriopathy and congenital or acquired heart disease. The presence of multiple risk factors may compound the stroke risk for some children (**Box 1**).[1]

Outcome
Clinical and radiological recurrence of AIS is seen in 10% to 30% of children.[1,8,9] The mortality rate from AIS is approximately 0.08 deaths per 100,000 children per year in the United States, with a higher mortality rate found in the Southeastern United States (referred to as the stroke belt) for reasons that remain unclear.[10] Despite the neural plasticity present in children, most children with stroke have persistent disability.

Risk factors
Arteriopathies Arteriopathies are the conditions most frequently associated with pediatric AIS and may be acute, transient, or progressive. Common arteriopathies include focal cerebral arteriopathy (FCA) of childhood, moyamoya, cervicocephalic arterial dissection, and sickle cell disease.[11]

Focal cerebral arteriopathy FCA is the term used by the IPSS group to describe an unexplained focal arterial stenosis in a child with AIS, including transient cerebral arteriopathy of childhood (TCA). In the IPSS, the only independent factor associated with FCA was recent upper respiratory tract infection.[12]

TCA is characterized by unilateral focal or segmental stenosis of the distal carotid arteries and proximal circle of Willis vessels. The stenosis may worsen for several months after the stroke but then stabilizes and can even improve by 6 months after the presentation.[13] AIS associated with TCA typically occurs in the distribution of the lenticulostriate branches of the proximal middle and anterior cerebral arteries. Antecedent viral infections may be found in some cases of TCA, although the exact cause is unknown. Possible causes include inflammation and vasculitis caused by infection or autoimmune disease, thromboembolic arterial occlusion or stenosis, intracranial dissection, arterial spasm, and prothrombotic factors.[13]

Postvaricella arteriopathy Varicella-associated AIS accounts for nearly one-third of childhood AIS. The most plausible mechanism is intraneuronal migration of the virus from the trigeminal ganglion along the trigeminal nerve to the cerebral arteries.[14] In a prospective study of children aged 6 months to 10 years with neuroimaging-confirmed AIS from 1992 to 1999 in Canada, 22 of 70 (31%) children with AIS had a varicella infection in the preceding year compared with 9% in the healthy population. The mean interval from varicella infection to AIS was 5.2 months. The presentation of varicella-associated strokes is less variable than nonvaricella-related AIS, with hemiparesis significantly more likely than seizures. Recurrent AIS occurred in 10 (45%) children in the varicella cohort compared with 8 (20%) children in the group without recent varicella.[14]

Additionally, children in the varicella cohort were more likely than children in the nonvaricella cohort to have an infarct located in the basal ganglia, limited to the anterior circulation, or stenosis of a large vessel. The vascular abnormalities in the varicella cohort consisted nearly exclusively of areas of stenosis in the proximal portion of the major cerebral arteries.[14]

Another study demonstrated that approximately one-third of children experience recurrent varicella-associated AIS up to 33 weeks after presentation despite antithrombotic prophylaxis.[15] Postvaricella arteriopathy generally takes a monophasic course with spontaneous regression of the stenosis. Occasionally, stenosis may progress for up to 6 months after stroke. AIS rarely recurs with antithrombotic prophylaxis after stenosis regression occurs, which suggests that AIS recurrence relates to acute vascular injury and thrombosis associated with the progression of vascular stenosis.[15]

Box 1
Risk factors for pediatric stroke

Cardiac

Congenital heart defects

Valvular heart disease

Right-to-left shunts

Cardiomyopathy

Endocarditis/myocarditis

Arrhythmia

Cardiac tumors

Cardiac surgery

Hematologic disorders and coagulopathies

Anemia

Sickle cell disease

Dehydration

Idiopathic Thrombocytopenia Purpura (ITP)/Thrombotic Thrombocytopenic Purpura (TTP)/ Hemolytic Uremic Syndrome (HUS)

Thrombocytosis

Polycythemia

Disseminated intravascular coagulation

Leukemia or other neoplasm

Congenital and acquired coagulation disorders

Pregnancy and the postpartum period

Vasculitis/Vasculopathies

Systemic lupus erythematosus

Polyarteritis nodosa

Takayasu arteritis

Kawasaki disease

Moyamoya syndrome/disease

Infection

Meningitis/encephalitis

Mastoiditis/otitis media

HIV

Varicella

Syphilis

Tuberculosis

Systemic infection

Metabolic/Miscellaneous

Homocystinuria

Fabry disease

Organic acidemia

Hyperlipidemia

Mitochondrial encephalopathy with lactic acidosis and strokelike episodes syndrome

Menkes disease

Other Vascular

Vasospasm (subarachnoid hemorrhage)

Migraine

Carotid ligation (eg, extracorporeal membrane oxygenation)

Fibromuscular dysplasia

Cervicocephalic arterial dissection

Arteriovenous malformation

Arteriography

Hereditary hemorrhagic telangiectasia

Sturge-Weber syndrome

Intracranial aneurysm

Trauma (including nonaccidental)

Blunt and penetrating cervical trauma

Brain tumor

Drugs

Cocaine

Amphetamines

Oral contraceptives

L-asparaginase

There are no specific accepted treatment protocols for varicella-associated stroke in children. The use of steroids or antiviral drugs is controversial and is not commented on by the American Heart Association (AHA) Stroke Council Guidelines. The prevention of varicella infection via vaccination will decrease the morbidity associated with postvaricella arteriopathy. Varicella vaccine contains live attenuated virus and was recommended in 1996 as a routine immunization for young children. A retrospective study of more than 3 million children found no association between varicella vaccine and ischemic stroke.[16]

Moyamoya disease and moyamoya syndrome Moyamoya syndrome is characterized by progressive stenosis of the distal intracranial internal carotid artery (ICA) and, less often, the proximal anterior cerebral artery (ACA), middle cerebral artery (MCA), basilar artery, and posterior cerebral artery. The term moyamoya is a Japanese word meaning "puff of smoke" and refers to the appearance of deep, fine, collateral vessels seen on conventional angiography. In the United States, the incidence is 0.086 per 100,000 children. All ethnic groups can be affected by moyamoya.[17]

Children with an associated medical condition are categorized as having moyamoya syndrome, whereas those with no known risk factors are said to have moyamoya disease. Moyamoya syndrome is seen in association with neurofibromatosis, Down syndrome, Williams syndrome, sickle cell disease, and after cranial irradiation.[1]

Moyamoya disease typically presents in children, with a peak incidence at 5 years of age. Recurrent transient ischemic attacks or ischemic strokes are common during childhood. Ischemic symptoms may be triggered by hyperventilation, crying, coughing, straining, or fever. Later in early adulthood, patients may more commonly suffer from intracranial hemorrhage.[17]

Absent flow voids in the ICA, MCA, and ACA coupled with abnormally prominent flow voids from basal ganglia and thalamic collateral vessels may be demonstrated on magnetic resonance angiography. These imaging findings are virtually diagnostic of moyamoya syndrome.[17]

Moyamoya disease results in recurrent strokes with gradual neurologic and cognitive deterioration in 50% to 60% of patients if untreated. Mortality rates of up to 4.3% are seen in moyamoya disease.[17] Surgical revascularization procedures are widely used for moyamoya syndrome, particularly for patients with cognitive decline or recurrent or progressive symptoms. Direct anastomosis procedures, most commonly a superficial temporal artery to MCA anastomosis, are often technically difficult to perform in children because of the small size of scalp donor vessels or MCA recipient vessels. For this reason, newer procedures, including encephaloduroarteriosynangiosis and encephalomyoarteriosynangiosis, have been developed for indirect bypass.[1]

A modification of the encephaloduroarteriosynangiosis procedure, called pial synangiosis, has been used with encouraging results. In this procedure, the superficial temporal artery is transposed and affixed to the brain surface to promote neovascularization. A review of 143 children with moyamoya syndrome treated with pial synangiosis demonstrated marked reductions in their stroke frequency after surgery. Although 67.8% had strokes preoperatively, 7.7% had strokes in the perioperative period and only 3.2% had strokes after at least 1 year of follow-up.[18] Potential complications of surgery for moyamoya include postoperative ischemic stroke, infection, spontaneous or traumatic subdural hematoma, and intracranial hemorrhage.[17]

Cervicocephalic arterial dissection Cervicocephalic arterial dissection (CCAD) is an underrecognized cause of stroke in children. A retrospective review of 213 children aged 1 month to 18 years with AIS who were included in the Canadian Pediatric Ischemic Stroke Registry from 1992 to 2002 demonstrated that CCAD accounts for 7.5% of children with AIS.[19] Warning symptoms, including headache, vomiting, dizziness, vertigo, diplopia, confusion, neck pain, and recurrent transient ischemic attacks, were present in 37.5% of those with CCAD. One-half had a history of head or neck trauma. The clinical presentation included headache (44%), altered consciousness (25%), seizures (12.5%), and focal deficits (87.5%).[19]

The predisposing factors for CCAD include trauma, connective tissue abnormalities, fibromuscular dysplasia, and anatomic variations. Migraine, infection, and hyperhomocysteinemia have also been considered risk factors. CCAD occurs both spontaneously and after blunt or penetrating trauma. Unlike adults, CCAD in children is most commonly found intracranially. Spontaneous anterior circulation arterial dissections (ACAD), in particular, tend to be intracranial, whereas posttraumatic ACAD is more often extracranial.[20]

High-resolution magnetic resonance imaging (MRI), with fat-saturated T1 imaging of the neck, and contrast-enhanced magnetic resonance angiography can help diagnose CCAD, although conventional angiography is the gold standard for diagnosis. Arteriographic features of CCAD include the presence of a string sign; double-lumen sign; short, smooth, tapered stenosis; and vessel occlusion of a parent arter.[1]

The recurrence rate of CCAD is about 1% per year.[1] Outcomes include complete recovery in 43%, mild to moderate deficits in 44%, and severe deficits in 13%. Follow-up angiography shows the resolution of abnormalities in 60% of vessels.[19]

The goal of therapy for CCAD is to prevent additional ischemic strokes until the vessel has healed. Options include immediate anticoagulation with intravenous unfractionated heparin (UFH) or low-molecular-weight heparin (LMWH) followed by a 3- to 6-month course of warfarin, continued LMWH, or platelet antiaggregant therapy. For patients who do not respond to medical management, proximal ligation, trapping procedures, and extracranial-intracranial bypass procedures have been attempted.[1]

SCD   SCD is one of the most common causes of childhood stroke, with a rate that is approximately 300 times higher than that seen in children without SCD.[21] Eleven percent of patients with SCD have a clinically apparent stroke by 20 years of age.[22] SCD contributes to stroke development because of the persistent endothelial injury from hypoxia, increased sheer stress, abnormal endothelial adherence of sickled red blood cells, and inflammation induced by reperfusion injury.[21] Stroke is a leading cause of death in children with SCD.[23]

The risk of stroke varies with the genotype. The Cooperative Study of Sickle Cell Disease (CSSCD) reported an age-adjusted incidence of first stroke of 0.61 per 100 patient-years in SCD hemoglobin SS (Hb SS), which is higher than that for hemoglobin SC (Hb SC), hemoglobin S-beta (+) thalassemia, and hemoglobin S-beta (0) thalassemia (0.15, 0.09, and 0.08, respectively, per 100 patient-years).[22] Among these first strokes, 54% were caused by cerebral infarction, 34% by intracranial hemorrhage, 11% by transient ischemic events, and 1% had features of both infarction and hemorrhage.[22] AIS is most common in children aged between 2 years and 9 years, whereas hemorrhagic stroke is most frequent in individuals aged between 20 and 29 years.[22]

In most cases of symptomatic stroke, infarction results from large vessel occlusion usually in the distribution of the distal ICA, proximal MCA, and ACA. Moyamoya syndrome, resulting from progressive narrowing of these vessels with compensatory collateral vessel development, occurs in about one-third of patients with stroke.[21] Children with this syndrome are at a higher risk of recurrent stroke, including hemorrhagic stroke caused by the rupture of moyamoya vessels or aneurysms. The site of bleeding may be subarachnoid, intraparenchymal, intraventricular, or a combination of these locations.[22]

With the availability of better imaging techniques, like MRI and angiography and transcranial Doppler, subtle subclinical injury to the brain caused by sickle cell-related vascular compromise has been demonstrated in approximately 20% of children with SCD.[21] The cause of these ischemic lesions is small vessel occlusion, mainly in arterial border zones. These lesions are known as silent infarcts because they are asymptomatic but appear as punctate lesions in the deep white matter of the brain on MRI. However, these lesions may not truly be silent because an increasing lesion burden correlates with significant neuropsychological deficits.[21]

Symptoms of AIS in SCD may include hemiparesis, dysphasia, gait disturbance, or altered consciousness. Children with SCD do not generally die acutely of AIS, although substantial morbidity may occur. In contrast, hemorrhagic stroke commonly presents with severe headache, vomiting, stiff neck, and altered consciousness. One-quarter to one-half of children with SCD will die within 2 weeks of a hemorrhagic stroke.[22]

The major identified risk factors for AIS with relative risks (RR) in the CSSCD are prior TIA (RR 56), low steady state hemoglobin (RR 1.9 per 1 g/dL decrease), rate of acute chest syndrome (RR 2.4 per event per year), episode of acute chest syndrome within the previous 2 weeks (RR 7.0), and elevated systolic blood pressure (RR 1.3 per 10 mm Hg increase).[22] The major risk factors identified for hemorrhagic stroke are low steady state hemoglobin (RR 1.6 per 1 g/dL decrease) and increased steady state leukocyte count (RR 1.9 per 5000/μL increase).[22]

TCD is an important tool in predicting the risk for stroke in children with SCD. It is a noninvasive procedure that measures the time-averaged mean velocity of blood flow in the large intracranial vessels, which is inversely related to arterial diameter. A focal increase in velocity usually suggests arterial stenosis. Because of their anemia, children with SCD generally have higher TCD flow velocities (130–140 cm/sec) than children without SCD (90 cm/sec).[24] In children with SCD, a mean velocity greater than 170 cm/sec is considered marginal, whereas values greater than 200 cm/sec in the middle cerebral or internal carotid artery are highly associated with an increased risk of stroke. The TCD can pick up abnormalities before lesions become evident on magnetic resonance angiography.[24] TCD has become part of routine screening for children with SCD. Children at a high risk for stroke on multiple studies should be started on a stroke-prevention protocol of chronic transfusion.[25]

The ability to identify patients with SCD at a high risk for stroke provides the opportunity to prevent a first stroke in children with SCD. The Stroke Prevention Trial in Sickle Cell Anemia (STOP I trial) included 130 children with SCD with no prior history of stroke and all had a blood flow velocity greater than 200 cm/sec on 2 repeated studies. The children were randomly assigned to observation or a chronic transfusion program with a goal HbS fraction of less than 30% of total hemoglobin. The trial was prematurely terminated because of a marked benefit in the prophylactic chronic transfusion group. There was one infarct in the transfusion group compared with 10 infarctions and one intracerebral hemorrhage in the control group.[26]

Once a patient starts a chronic transfusion protocol, stopping it results in a reversion back to a high risk for stroke. This point was demonstrated in the STOP II Trial, which was similarly terminated early when a significant number of patients who stopped receiving chronic transfusion reverted to a high risk of stroke and 2 patients had a stroke. There were no strokes or reversion to high stroke risk in the patients assigned to continue transfusion.[27]

For those children with SCD presenting acutely with ischemic stroke, urgent transfusion therapy followed by immediate exchange transfusion to achieve a HbS fraction of less than 30% and hemoglobin level of approximately 10 g/dL is recommended (**Box 2**). Initial treatment also involves administering intravenous normotonic fluids to prevent dehydration. Early consultation with the hematology department is important to determine the best protocol to follow regarding hydration and transfusion. After the acute episode, these children should be treated with chronic transfusion therapy to prevent stroke recurrence, which occurs in approximately two-thirds of patients within 2 years of the initial stroke.[21,25]

At this time, no effective alternative to chronic transfusion therapy is available. Special care should be taken to minimize the adverse consequences of transfusion, which include iron overload, alloimmunization, and infection.[25] Hydroxyurea, the only Food and Drug Administration–approved drug for treating SCD, failed to show effectiveness in preventing stroke recurrence in a large multicenter trial (Stroke With Transfusions Changing to Hydroxyurea [SWiTCH] trial).[28]

Box 2
Acute management of ischemic stroke in children with SCD

- Hydration
- Urgent transfusion therapy followed by immediate exchange transfusion
- Goal HbS fraction of less than 30% and hemoglobin level of approximately 10 g/dL
- Initiation of chronic transfusion protocol to prevent stroke recurrence

Angiography should be considered carefully in all patients with SCD because angiography might promote sickling. The treatment of subarachnoid hemorrhage in children with SCD involves administering intravenous normotonic fluids to prevent dehydration. In adults, nimodepine, a calcium antagonist that improves outcomes by counteracting delayed arterial vasospasm, is indicated; the use in this setting in young children is not approved but is reasonable on an empiric basis. The adult dosage of 60 mg orally every 4 hours should be adjusted for weight. Aneurysms may be repaired when possible, either surgically or endovascularly. In children with SCD and moyamoya syndrome, surgical treatment has been used to restore the circulation of the ischemic brain area, thereby reducing the risk of ischemic stroke.[25]

Cardiac disease One-fourth to one-third of AIS in children results from cardiac disease.[1,7] Most of these occur in children already known to have a cardiac lesion at the time of their stroke. Stroke has been described with most types of cardiac lesions, although complex congenital heart lesions with right-to-left shunting and cyanosis (eg, atrial or ventricular septal defects with pulmonary hypertension) are particularly prone to cause stroke. Children with heart disease who have a low hemoglobin concentration resulting from iron deficiency seem to have a higher risk of arterial stroke. In contrast, those with a markedly elevated hematocrit may be at more risk for cerebral venous sinus thrombosis.[1] The significance of a patent foramen ovale (PFO) in a child with stroke is uncertain and finding one on diagnostic echocardiogram should not exclude further etiologic investigation.[1] Children can develop a stroke as a result of acquired disorders of the myocardium or cardiac valves. Infective endocarditis involving the left side of the heart increases the risk of stroke.[1] Although cardiac arrhythmias are an uncommon cause of stroke in children, specific types of arrhythmias have been described in children with stroke. Cardiomyopathy or myocardial infarction from various causes can lead to cardiac arrhythmia or decreased left ventricular wall motion predisposing to cerebral embolism.[1] Cardiomyopathy can occur with mitochondrial disorders, various forms of muscular dystrophy, Friedreich ataxia, some congenital myopathies, and Fabry disease. Myocardial infarction in children most often occurs in the setting of childhood polyarteritis nodosa, homozygous type II hyperlipoproteinemia, or Kawasaki disease.[1] Congestive heart failure with reduced ejection fraction increases the risk of embolism. The risk of stroke is increased for children receiving extracorporeal membrane oxygenation (ECMO).[1] Intracranial bleeds and infarction may be caused by ligation of the carotid artery and internal jugular vein, systemic heparinization, thrombocytopenia, coagulopathies, or systolic hypertension. The long-term risks of ligation of the carotid artery are not known, so an increased risk of stroke may occur as the person ages. Venous-venous (VV) ECMO does not require tying off the carotid artery. Although this may prove to have fewer risks, not all people are candidates for VV ECMO. Thromboembolic stroke can complicate cardiac catheterization and cardiac surgery. A study from the Hospital for Sick Children in Toronto found that among 5526 children less than 18 years of age with congenital heart disease who underwent cardiac surgery, the risk for AIS/CVST was 5.4 strokes per 1000 children.[29]

Anticoagulation is recommended for those children who are thought to have a high risk of embolism from cardiac disease. Surgical repair or transcatheter closure is indicated for major atrial septal defects, both to reduce the stroke risk and to prevent long-term cardiac complications.[1]

Hypercoagulable disorders One or more prothrombotic states have been identified in 20% to 50% of children presenting with AIS.[30] The presence of a prothrombotic state is often combined with other mechanisms for thrombotic vascular occlusion and is rarely an isolated cause.[30] Children with other risk factors for stroke who also have a hypercoagulable disorder are at the highest risk for stroke.

Prothrombotic abnormalities reduce the threshold for the development of thrombosis and may be important in the pathogenesis of childhood AIS. It is valuable to identify a prothrombotic abnormality in children with AIS to provide appropriate treatment, prevent recurrences, and provide information on the risk of thrombosis in family members.[31]

In some cases, the abnormality is inherited, such as the deficiencies of coagulation inhibitors or increased activity of coagulation proteins. A recent meta-analysis of 22 observational studies that included 1526 children with AIS, 238 with cerebral venous sinus thrombosis, and 2799 control subjects, estimated the impact of thrombophilia on the risk of first childhood stroke. The highest odds ratios (OR) were found for combined genetic traits, deficiency of protein C, the presence of antiphospholipid antibodies, and elevated lipoprotein (a) (**Table 1**).[32]

Screening for inherited thrombophilia in children should be done under the guidance of a pediatric hematologist. Many of the tests are time sensitive, and interpreting the results of the screening tests can be challenging because of the variability of normative reference values in children.

In some children, acquired thrombophilia caused by underlying illness may lead to stroke such as occurs in systemic lupus erythematosus, hemolytic uremic syndrome, thrombotic thrombocytopenic purpura, malignancy, nephrotic syndrome, paroxysmal nocturnal hemoglobinuria, polycythemia rubra vera, essential thrombocythemia, and disseminated intravascular coagulation. Homocystinuria is an uncommon but well-recognized cause of both arterial and venous occlusion. Medications, including L-asparaginase and oral contraceptives, may be prothrombotic.[1]

Pregnancy is a stroke risk factor in adolescent girls. Alterations of multiple coagulation factors occur during pregnancy. The risk of both brain infarction (usually venous) and hemorrhage is increased during the 6 weeks after delivery but not during pregnancy. Although the incidence is low, ischemic stroke and intracranial hemorrhage account for at least 4.0% to 8.5% of maternal mortality in the United States. Eclampsia remains the leading cause of both hemorrhagic and nonhemorrhagic stroke.[1]

Iron deficiency anemia Previously healthy children with stroke are 10 times more likely to have iron deficiency anemia (IDA) than healthy children without stroke. Several studies suggest that IDA is a significant risk factor for stroke in otherwise healthy

Table 1 Prothrombotic conditions associated with pediatric AIS	
Condition	OR (CI)
Two or more genetic thrombophilias	18.8 (95% 6.5–54.1)
Protein C deficiency	11.0 (95% 5.1–23.6)
Antiphospholipid antibodies/lupus anticoagulant	7.0 (95% 3.7–13.1)
Elevated lipoprotein (a)	6.5 (95% 4.5–9.6)
Factor V Leiden mutation G1691A	3.7 (95% 2.8–4.9)
Factor II G20210A (prothrombin) mutation	2.6 (95% 1.7–4.1)
MTHFR TT genotype	1.6 (95% 1.2–2.1)

Abbreviations: CI, confidence interval; MTHFR, methylenetetrahydrafolate reductase T677T.
Data from Kenet G, Lütkhoff LK, Albisetti M, et al. Impact of thrombophilia on risk of arterial ischemic stroke or cerebral sinovenous thrombosis in neonates and children: a systematic review and meta-analysis of observational studies. Circulation 2010;121(16):1838–47.

children.[33,34] Several theories have been proposed to explain this finding: a hypercoagulable state directly related to iron deficiency or anemia, thrombocytosis secondary to IDA, and anemic hypoxia whereby a mismatch of oxygen supply and demand leads to ischemia and infarction.[33,35]

Vasculitis Primary vasculitides associated with stroke include Takayasu arteritis, giant cell arteritis, polyarteritis nodosa, Kawasaki disease, and primary angiitis of the central nervous system (CNS). Secondary vasculitides are associated with collagen vascular diseases, like lupus or infections. Bacterial meningitis; viral infections, including HIV, varicella, syphilis, and CNS tuberculosis; and fungal infections can cause cerebral vasculitides resulting in stroke. CNS infections, such as meningitis and encephalitis, are associated with up to 10% of all childhood AIS.[1] Vascular inflammation, thrombosis caused by reduced cerebral perfusion in systemic hypotension, raised intracranial pressure, and low cerebrospinal fluid glucose may all contribute to stroke pathophysiology. Hypotension and hypercoagulability secondary to bacteremia or sepsis can lead to AIS.[1]

Metabolic Several metabolic conditions are associated with AIS by affecting changes in the wall of the cerebral vessels. These conditions include cerebral autosomal-dominant arteriopathy with subcortical infarcts and leukoencephalopathy, Fabry disease, Homocystinuria, and Menkes disease.

Some metabolic conditions are associated with metabolic stroke rather than arterial stroke: the syndrome of mitochondrial encephalopathy with lactic acidosis and stroke-like episodes, organic acidemias (eg, methylmalonic, propionic, isovaleric), and urea cycle disorders. These metabolic strokes may be associated with systemic illness, persistent vomiting, hypoglycemia, or diabetes.[1]

Acute management of pediatric arterial ischemic stroke
The goals of acute management in pediatric stroke are to preserve neurologic function, limit the extension of the area of infarction, and prevent early recurrent thromboembolic events. Beyond the acute phase, secondary preventative measures are of the utmost importance given the 10% to 30% recurrence rate of stroke in children.[9]

Evidence-based decision making in pediatric AIS is hampered by the lack of randomized controlled data. The current recommendations discussed here reflect the official guidelines from the American Heart Association Stroke Council, the Council on Cardiovascular Disease in the Young, and the American College of Chest Physicians (ACCP).[1,36] These recommendations (**Box 3**) are based on reviews of less-rigorous studies in the literature, expert opinion, and extrapolation from adult studies.

Box 3
Acute treatment of AIS

1. The initial therapy should be instituted with UFH/LMWH until dissection and embolic causes are excluded (AHA Stroke Council recommendation).

2. Aspirin may be an acceptable alternative at a dosage of 1 to 5 mg/kg/d (ACCP).

3. Thrombolysis cannot be endorsed for the treatment of AIS in children outside of clinical trials.

4. The treatment of adolescents who otherwise meet criteria for tissue plasminogen activator is debatable and should be considered on a case-by-case basis with consultation with a neurologist at a tertiary care center. Strict protocol needs to be followed to prevent ICH.

5. The phone number, 1-800-NOCLOTS, may be useful for consultation.

However, it should be emphasized that ischemic stroke in children is fundamentally a different illness than stroke in older adults. The mechanism of thrombus formation in adults is more commonly associated with atherosclerosis-driven platelet activation, whereas illnesses leading to fibrin clot formation are more often responsible for stroke in children. Therefore, the results of antithrombotic trials in adults are not so easily transferable to children.

Unlike adult patients, UFH or LMWH may be initiated for children with acute ischemic stroke pending evaluation of the stroke cause. Children are much more likely to suffer an AIS secondary to cervical artery dissections, vasculopathy, heritable coagulopathies, or nonatherosclerotic cardiac disease. The recommended fist-line therapy for all of these conditions is anticoagulation.[9] For children with SCD or Moyamoya disease, the initial treatment with UFH or LMWH is not indicated.[1,36] Anticoagulation in childhood AIS seems to be safe.[37]

Aspirin and related antiplatelet medications are the mainstay of secondary prevention in adults with AIS but require different consideration in children. Nonrandomized studies have found differing results as to the efficacy of antiplatelet versus anticoagulants for secondary prevention. No randomized trials of antithrombotic use in children for the management of stroke have been conducted. However, studies have demonstrated that treatment with either antithrombotic is superior to no treatment.[38,39] Dosing recommendations for aspirin are 3 to 5 mg/kg/d, with reduction to 1 to 3 mg/kg/d if gastric distress or bleeding occurs.[1,36] Plavix (clopidogrel) may be considered in children with aspirin intolerance or aspirin failure.[1]

Although there are numerous case reports of the successful use of thrombolytics, such as tissue plasminogen activator (tPA) in children with AIS, reliable multicenter randomized controlled data are lacking. There are limited published safety and efficacy data regarding the use of thrombolytics in children.[40,41] For this reason, the AHA Stroke Council and the ACCP do not currently recommend the use of tPA outside of a clinical trial.[1,36] An international multicenter clinical trial (Thrombolysis in Pediatric Stroke) examining safety, dosage, and feasibility of thrombolytics is currently underway.[42]

A gray area exists regarding the use of tPA in adolescent patients who otherwise meet the standard adult tPA eligibility criteria. There is no consensus about the use of tPA in adolescents or a commonly accepted definition as to what age defines adolescence in this circumstance. All guidelines and published data demonstrate that if thrombolytics are to be given, clinicians must adhere to standard adult protocols with regard to the dosage and the timing of therapy. Delays in administration from the onset of stroke past the accepted time ranges are likely to result in unacceptable risks of hemorrhage.[40,43]

For guidance, a pediatric stroke consultation service has been established (1-800-NOCLOTS). The telephone line is based at the Hospital for Sick Children in Toronto and is staffed by pediatric hematologists and neurologists.[44]

Supportive neuroprotective measures are important for the preservation of neurologic function and limitation of the ischemic penumbra (**Box 4**). Supplemental oxygen is recommended only when patients are hypoxemic and has not shown to be beneficial in those who are normoxemic.[1,45] Fever may worsen the degree of brain damage after AIS and should, therefore, be controlled with antipyretics. There are limited data on the role of induced hypothermia in adult patients, and there is not enough information to recommend therapeutic brain cooling for pediatric patients with stroke.[46,47] The treatment of dehydration, anemia, and hyperglycemia are recommended. In adult AIS, permissive hypertension is recommended in all but the most severe blood pressures (>220 mm Hg systolic blood pressure or >120 mm Hg diastolic blood pressure). There

---

Box 4
Supportive neuroprotective measures

1. Provide supplemental oxygenation only for patients who are hypoxemic. There is no role for hyperbaric oxygen except in decompression sickness or air embolism.

2. There is no empiric treatment of seizures.

3. Provide adequate hydration with normotonic solutions.

4. Provide normalization of serum glucose.

5. There is permissive hypertension in the acute period unless anticoagulation is to be initiated.

6. Anemia should be treated.

7. Treat fever with antipyretics.

8. Although brain cooling is an appropriate treatment in neonates with hypoxic-ischemic encephalopathy, there is no role in pediatric stroke for therapeutic hypothermia outside of clinical trials.

9. There should be early consultation with neurosurgery if there is a high suspicion for increased intracranial pressure warranting the consideration of decompression.

---

are no consensus guidelines addressing permissive hypertension specifically in children, but it seems rational to control excessive hypertension particularly when anticoagulant medications are being administered. Antiepileptic drugs are only recommended in patients with clinical or electrographic seizures.[1] The treatment of increased intracranial pressure in children is similar to therapies used in adults. Neurosurgery should be consulted early for consideration of decompressive surgery if there is a concern for increased intracranial pressure.

Perinatal Ischemic Stroke

Perinatal stroke refers to cerebrovascular events that occur between 20 weeks of fetal life and 28 days after birth. As in older children, strokes in neonates may be AIS, hemorrhagic, or CVST (which can cause both infarction and hemorrhage).[48] AIS is more common in the perinatal period than hemorrhagic strokes, representing approximately 80% of strokes, and may be caused by arterial occlusion, hypoperfusion in watershed territories, or venous outflow obstruction.

Epidemiology

The incidence of perinatal AIS is 10 times greater than that of childhood stroke and ranks second only to the ischemic strokes in the elderly population. Because of the lack of prospective studies on the incidence of perinatal strokes, estimates are based on retrospective cohort studies. The annual incidence of perinatal AIS is 29 per 100,000 live births or 1 per 3500.[2]

Presentation

Unlike older children and adults, the clinical presentation of neonates with cerebral infarction can be subtle and nonspecific. Seizures are the presenting symptom in 85% to 90% of infants with perinatal AIS[49] and may be clonic, tonic, or focal (typically contralateral to the affected hemisphere in unilateral cerebral infarction). Seizure onset from AIS typically occurs on the first day of life, with 90% presenting within the first 3 days of life. Perinatal AIS is diagnosed in 10% to 15% of neonates with seizures.[49]

Most cases of AIS result from arterial infarction in the distribution of the MCA. Therefore, the arm and face are likely to be more affected than the leg.[50] Infants with unilateral lesions may have a hemiparesis but this can be difficult to detect in infancy. It may appear as asymmetry of spontaneous movements. Mild quadriparesis in the case of bilateral brain lesions is usually not detected until late infancy. Other presentations may include apnea, lethargy, and poor feeding.[48,49]

Cause

The causes of perinatal AIS can be embolic from cardiac origin, thrombotic from disturbed hemostasis, or related to disorders of the cerebral arteries. These disorders may originate from maternal, placental, or fetal/neonatal conditions alone or in combination. Newborns are at risk for emboli to cerebral vessels from thrombosis of placental vessels that may lead to emboli being released into the fetal circulation as the placenta separates at birth. Additionally, venous clots can pass through the PFO and proceed to the cerebral vessels. Other right-to-left shunts can occur in the presence of congenital heart disease. Emboli can also be a result of iatrogenic causes, such as indwelling umbilical vessel catheters.[48]

Coagulation disorders, which have been identified in half of the infants and children with stroke, may be an even greater risk factor in newborns. Inherited prothrombotic disorders that are probable risk factors for perinatal AIS include antiphospholipid antibodies/lupus anticoagulant; factor V Leiden; congenital deficiency of proteins C, S, or antithrombin; increased lipoprotein (a); prothrombin gene mutation; and methylenetetrahydrafolate reductase T677T genotype (MTHFR).[48]

Evaluation

Following a thorough examination and neurologic assessment, the evaluation of a neonate with suspected stroke should include a complete blood count with differential blood and cerebrospinal fluid analysis with cultures, serum electrolyte analysis, and urine toxicology screening. For persistent seizures, studies to detect inborn errors of metabolism should be considered. Herpes encephalitis may have a similar presentation and, if suspected, antiviral therapy should be started and continued until all relevant tests prove normal.[50]

In cases of confirmed infarction, further evaluation includes a cardiac echo to exclude an underlying cardiac abnormality as well as an amplitude integrated electroencephalogram (aEEG) or full EEG. Confirmation of normal clotting status is needed early; although genetic prothrombotic disorders may be tested for at any time, protein-based assays should be performed soon after symptom onset and repeated 3 to 6 months later if abnormal. A detailed maternal, family, pregnancy, and delivery history should be taken and, if possible, placental assessment should be performed.[50]

Outcome

Long-term disabilities after a perinatal stroke include cognitive and sensory impairments, cerebral palsy, and epilepsy.[49,50] The recurrence risk for cerebral events after perinatal AIS is low, roughly 1% to 8%.[1,49] Factors associated with an increased recurrence rate include thrombophilic states and comorbidities, such as congenital heart disease or dehydration. Unilateral AIS is not associated with an increased mortality unless there are other complicating conditions.[50]

Treatment

In the acute phase of perinatal AIS, supportive measures, such as the maintenance of normal hydration, temperature, electrolyte, hematologic, oxygenation, and acid-base status are recommended. Anticonvulsants may be given along with antibiotics or antivirals if sepsis is suspected.[50] Randomized controlled trials addressing the acute or chronic treatment of perinatal stroke are not available. The ACCP recommends the administration of UFH or LMWH in neonates with a first AIS only if an ongoing cardi-oembolic source can be documented. The AHA Stroke Council also recommends UFH or LMWH in severe thrombophilias.[1] Otherwise, anticoagulation or antiplatelet therapy is not recommended in neonatal stroke because the risk of recurrent stroke is low and the lesion is not thought to extend further by the time the diagnosis is made.

Hemorrhagic Transformation of Pediatric AIS

There are limited data available regarding hemorrhagic transformation of AIS in chil-dren. It may occur within 30 days of symptom onset in 30% of children and is mostly asymptomatic. It has been shown to occur less frequently in children with vasculop-athy as the cause of AIS and has not been associated with anticoagulation versus anti-platelet therapy. Similar to adults, larger infarct volume may be associated with hemorrhagic transformation and worse outcome.[51]

CVST

CVST is a rare but important form of stroke that results from thrombosis of the dural venous sinuses, which drain blood from the brain. The incidence of childhood CVST is 0.67 per 100,000 children per year from term birth to 18 years of age, with neonates composing 43% of the patients.[52] Venous congestion can lead to both parenchymal ischemia and hemorrhage. Subarachnoid and subdural hemorrhages are less frequent. The superficial venous system is more frequently involved than the deep system, and the most common sites of CVST are the transverse, superior sagittal, sigmoid, and straight sinuses.[53]

CVST in Neonates

Neonatal CVST presents similarly to perinatal AIS (see section on perinatal AIS presentation). It may arise because of damage to cerebral sinus structures caused by molding of the cranium from birth or from placental lesions that may lead to an inflammatory and prothrombotic state in the placenta and fetus.[50] Neonates also have reduced levels of circulating anticoagulant proteins and relative dehydration and hemoconcentration, which could also lead to a prothrombotic state.[54] Prothrom-botic states have been identified in 20% of neonates with CVST.

Risk factors
Perinatal complications (51%) and dehydration (30%) were the most frequent illnesses found in 69 neonates with CVST in the Canadian Pediatric Ischemic Stroke Registry. The perinatal complications included hypoxia at birth, premature rupture of mem-branes, maternal infection, placental abruption, and gestational diabetes.[52]

Outcome
Among neonates with CVST, neurologic deficits have been observed in 28% to 83% of patients. Studies have demonstrated a mortality rate of 7% to 8%.[54]

Treatment
The role of anticoagulation in neonatal CVST is controversial because recurrent CVST is rare. However, the extension of the initial thrombus in the week following diagnosis occurs less often in neonates on anticoagulation therapy compared with those not treated with anticoagulation.[55] The ACCP and the AHA Stroke Council guidelines recommend treatment of neonates with CVST without significant intracranial hemor-rhage using UFH or LMWH initially, followed by LMWH or warfarin for 6 to 12 weeks.[1] For neonates with CVST and significant hemorrhage, radiological monitoring is

recommended with commencement of anticoagulation therapy if extension of the thrombus occurs 5 to 7 days after the initial hemorrhage.[50] The safety of anticoagulation in neonates is yet to be fully studied. However, in a small study of 10 neonates with CVST and unilateral thalamic hemorrhage, 7 were treated with LMWH without any side effects.[56]

CVST in Infants and Older Children

Presentation
The clinical manifestations of CVST in children are subtle and nonspecific. An altered level of consciousness and encephalopathy, focal neurologic deficits (cranial nerve palsies, hemiparesis, hemisensory loss), and diffuse neurologic symptoms (headache, nausea, emesis) may result. Focal and diffuse neurologic signs are more common in older infants and children than seizures.[52]

Risk factors
The conditions that are associated with CVST in children outside of the neonatal period include common childhood illnesses, such as fever, infection, and anemia, and medical conditions, such as congenital heart disease, nephrotic syndrome, systemic lupus erythematosus, and malignancy. Otitis media and mastoiditis, meningitis, head trauma, and recent intracranial surgery are strongly associated with CVST. Prothrombotic states have been identified in 24% to 64% of children with CVST.[53] Dehydration is another important risk factor for pediatric CVST, which can be caused by increased fluid loss or poor oral intake.[53]

Outcome
CVST-specific mortality is less than 10%, but motor and cognitive sequelae may require long-term rehabilitative regimens. Between 10% and 20% of children who have CVST will experience a recurrent symptomatic venous event, at least half of which are systemic rather than cerebral.[53]

Treatment
Many infants and older children receive anticoagulation in the acute setting with UFH or LMWH or oral warfarin. This regimen is often followed by chronic anticoagulation with LMWH or warfarin for 3 to 6 months. There are no randomized data on thrombolysis, thrombectomy, or surgical decompression for CVST.[53]

HEMORRHAGIC STROKE
Presentation
Children younger than 6 years of age with hemorrhagic stroke are more likely to present with altered mental status and seizures, whereas older children more commonly present with headache and focal neurologic signs. The typical pattern of presentation is the abrupt onset of clinical signs followed by progressive neurologic deterioration.[57]

Cause
Childhood hemorrhagic stroke, which includes spontaneous intraparenchymal and nontraumatic subarachnoid hemorrhages, accounts for approximately half of all childhood strokes. It tends to be associated with intracranial vascular anomalies (48%) or medical disorders, such as hematologic abnormalities (10%–30%) or brain tumors (9%), whereas in a significant minority of children, no identifiable cause is identified (19%).[57]

Intracranial vascular anomalies include arteriovenous malformations, aneurysms, and cavernous malformations. Hematologic causes of intraparenchymal hemorrhage include thrombocytopenia, hemophilia, von Willebrand disease, and coagulopathy secondary to hepatic dysfunction or vitamin K deficiency. Brain hemorrhage is estimated to occur in 0.1% to 1.0% of children with idiopathic thrombocytopenia purpura and in 2.9% to 12.0% of children with hemophilia. Hemorrhagic stroke in the context of SCD is common, as described previously in this article.[58]

Hemorrhagic Stroke in Neonates

Hemorrhagic stroke in the perinatal period can occur from conversion of ischemic infarction of arterial or venous origin or via intraparenchymal hemorrhage from vascular anomalies or bleeding diatheses. In a retrospective study from 1993 to 2003 in California, 20 cases of perinatal hemorrhagic stroke were described. The rate of perinatal hemorrhagic stroke in this population was 6.2 per 100,000 live births.[59] All of these patients presented with encephalopathy; 65% had seizures and 5% had focal weakness. Nineteen of the 20 were intracerebral hemorrhages and one was a subarachnoid hemorrhage. No causes for hemorrhage were identified in 15 patients. Four patients had thrombocytopenia and one had a cavernous malformation as the cause. Predictors of perinatal hemorrhage included fetal distress, emergency caesarian section delivery, prematurity, and postmaturity. Birth weight was not found to be a predictor. Neonates with a history of ECMO, coarctation of the aorta, and venous thrombosis are also at risk for hemorrhagic stroke.[59]

Outcome

Hemorrhagic stroke has a higher mortality than AIS. Limited data exist on outcomes. Studies have shown that the ratio of hemorrhage volume to brain volume positively correlates with increasing disability and poorer quality of life. Initial Glasgow Coma Score, hemorrhage location, and ventricular involvement do not seem to predict outcomes.[57]

Approximately one-third of children have a good outcome with little impairment, another third have deficits that range from moderate to severe, and one-third die of acute hemorrhage, recurring hemorrhage, or from an underlying disorder. Very few children develop epilepsy.[57]

The 5-year cumulative recurrence rate for hemorrhage is approximately 10%.[60] To prevent recurrence in children with intracranial vascular anomalies, the anomalies should be corrected when possible. Microsurgery, radiosurgery, and embolization are among the treatment options.

Treatment

A child with acute hemorrhagic stroke should be monitored in a pediatric intensive care unit. Although an awake patient can be monitored noninvasively, those children who demonstrate significant alteration of mental status should have intracranial pressure monitoring with the measurement of cerebral perfusion pressure.[60]

Children should neither be given hypotonic fluids nor be allowed to take anything by mouth to prevent cerebral edema and aspiration respectively. Blood pressure, body temperature, and blood sugar should be kept in the normal range for age. Neurologic examinations to check for signs of increased intracranial pressure and herniation should be conducted frequently. Some patients will require interventions, such as hyperosmotic treatments for elevated intracranial pressure or surgical management.[60]

Repeat computed tomography (CT) scans to look for hydrocephalus, extension of intracerebral hematoma, herniation, or vasospasm, in cases of subarachnoid hemorrhage, may be needed if further deterioration occurs. Patients who have cardiopulmonary compromise may need ventilatory or circulatory support.[60] If patients have a known disorder of hemostasis, specific treatment to address this disorder is needed. Patients may also require medications to control seizures.[57]

DIFFERENTIAL DIAGNOSIS OF PEDIATRIC STROKE

The differential diagnosis of pediatric stroke is broad because numerous other conditions can present with acute neurologic deficits (**Box 5**).[61]

DIAGNOSTIC EVALUATION OF CHILDREN WITH SUSPECTED STROKE

Children who are suspected of having a stroke should undergo urgent neuroimaging (**Box 6**). If neuroimaging is not immediately available, consideration should be given to transferring the child to a hospital with neuroimaging and neurosurgical and intensive care capabilities. The least invasive study that will provide an adequate assessment is usually the test to perform. If immediately available, general consensus is that MRI is an ideal method to evaluate neonates, infants, and children with suspected stroke.[1]

MRI studies should include sequences to detect hemorrhage, delineate anatomy, characterize focal lesions, and determine if a stroke is acute, subacute, or chronic. These studies may include T1, T2, fluid-attenuated inversion recovery (FLAIR), and diffusion-weighted imaging (DWI) sequences.[1]

The temporal evolution of diffusion abnormalities on MRI is distinct in neonates compared with older children and adults. DWI may underestimate the extent of infarct during the first 24 hours and after day 5 in neonates. T2 and FLAIR MRI sequences are more reliable than diffusion at day 7 and later in term newborns.[62]

Box 5
Conditions that mimic stroke in children

Brain tumor

Structural brain lesions

Prolonged postictal paralysis (Todd)

Migraine

Familial alternating hemiplegia

Metabolic stroke

Idiopathic intracranial hypertension

Intracranial infection (brain abscess, meningoencephalitis), acute disseminated encephalomyelitis

Reversible posterior leukoencephalopathy syndrome

Postinfectious cerebellitis

Musculoskeletal conditions

Nonaccidental trauma

Drug toxicity

Psychogenic conditions

Data from Shellhaas RA, Smith SE, O'Tool E, et al. Mimics of childhood stroke: characteristics of a prospective cohort. Pediatrics 2006;118(2):704–9.

Box 7
Studies to consider in the evaluation of children with acute stroke

Brain imaging

Electrocardiogram/echocardiogram

Complete blood count

Coagulation studies

Fibrinogen

Erythrocyte sedimentation rate

Serum electrolytes

Hepatic transaminases

Coagulability studies (with hematology consultation)

Hemoglobin electrophoresis

Cholesterol and triglycerides

Serum amino acids/urine organic acids

Toxicology screen

Pregnancy test (adolescent girls)

Lactate

Lumbar puncture (consider with caution if risk of herniation)

---

pacemakers, or other contraindications to MRI are best evaluated with CT. CT angiography and venography may also be performed.[1]

Cranial ultrasound is used routinely for neonatal imaging and can be performed until the closure of the anterior fontanelle. Although ultrasound is often used to detect intraventricular hemorrhage and periventricular leukomalacia, it is less sensitive than CT and MRI in the detection of cerebral ischemic lesions. CVST is a difficult diagnosis to confirm with ultrasound. Ultrasound imaging of the posterior fossa is also limited.[1]

CA can establish the cause of stroke in most children but is the most invasive of imaging options.[58] Most children require general anesthesia to undergo CA. During the first year of life, the risk of CA is increased because of the small size of the vascular tree, so the decision to perform angiography in these younger patients must be weighed carefully. In many instances, MRA or CT angiography will suffice in these patients. Diagnostic CA may need to be done in concert with therapeutic endovascular procedures even in this very young population.[63]

There are no guidelines addressing laboratory or ancillary testing for the assessment of pediatric stroke (**Box 7**). Tests to look for specific causes of stroke, such as coagulopathies, cardiac disease, or hematological disorders, should be considered with guidance from multidisciplinary consultation with pediatric hematologists, neurologists, radiologists, and any other relevant specialists.

SUMMARY

Pediatric stroke is a rare but important entity. There are age-specific differences in the causes, manifestations, and treatment of stroke in children of which ED physicians need to be aware to ensure prompt diagnosis and treatment of children with stroke syndromes. Although large clinical trials are difficult to conduct in children with stroke because of its low incidence and heterogeneity of causes, continued research and additional experience are needed. Randomized controlled trials are needed to establish the safety and efficacy of acute and preventative treatments of pediatric stroke. It is clear from a review of the literature on stroke in children that merely applying our knowledge of stroke in adults to children with stroke is insufficient.

REFERENCES

1. Roach ES, Golomb MR, Adams R, et al. Management of stroke in infants and children: a scientific statement from a Special Writing Group of the American Heart Association Stroke Council and the Council on Cardiovascular Disease in the Young. Stroke 2008;39(9):2644–91.
2. Agrawal N, Johnston SC, Wu YW, et al. Imaging data reveal a higher pediatric stroke incidence than prior US estimates. Stroke 2009;40(11):3415–21.
3. Fullerton HJ, Wu YW, Zhao S, et al. Risk of stroke in children: ethnic and gender disparities. Neurology 2003;61(2):189–94.
4. Golomb MR, Fullerton HJ, Nowak-Gottl U, et al. Male predominance in childhood ischemic stroke: findings from the international pediatric stroke study. Stroke 2009;40(1):52–7.
5. Rafay MF, Pontigon AM, Chiang J, et al. Delay to diagnosis in acute pediatric arterial ischemic stroke. Stroke 2009;40(1):58–64.
6. Zimmer JA, Garg BP, Williams LS, et al. Age-related variation in presenting signs of childhood arterial ischemic stroke. Pediatr Neurol 2007;37(3):171–5.
7. Mackay MT, Wiznitzer M, Benedict SL, et al. Arterial ischemic stroke risk factors: the International Pediatric Stroke Study. Ann Neurol 2011;69(1):130–40.
8. Fullerton HJ, Wu YW, Sidney S, et al. Risk of recurrent childhood arterial ischemic stroke in a population-based cohort: the importance of cerebrovascular imaging. Pediatrics 2007;119(3):495–501.
9. Goldenberg NA, Bernard TJ, Fullerton HJ, et al. Antithrombotic treatments, outcomes, and prognostic factors in acute childhood-onset arterial ischaemic stroke: a multicentre, observational, cohort study. Lancet Neurol 2009;8(12):1120–7.
10. Fullerton HJ, Elkins JS, Johnston SC. Pediatric stroke belt: geographic variation in stroke mortality in US children. Stroke 2004;35(7):1570–3.
11. Fox CK, Fullerton HJ. Recent advances in childhood arterial ischemic stroke. Curr Atheroscler Rep 2010;12(4):217–24.
12. Amlie-Lefond C, Bernard TJ, Sébire G, et al. Predictors of cerebral arteriopathy in children with arterial ischemic stroke: results of the International Pediatric Stroke Study. Circulation 2009;119(10):1417–23.
13. Chabrier S, Rodesch G, Lasjaunias P, et al. Transient cerebral arteriopathy: a disorder recognized by serial angiograms in children with stroke. J Child Neurol 1998;13(1):27–32.
14. Askalan R, Laughlin S, Mayank S, et al. Chickenpox and stroke in childhood: a study of frequency and causation. Stroke 2001;32(6):1257–62.
15. Lanthier S, Armstrong D, Domi T, et al. Post-varicella arteriopathy of childhood: natural history of vascular stenosis. Neurology 2005;64(4):660–3.
16. Donahue JG, Kieke BA, Yih WK, et al. Varicella vaccination and ischemic stroke in children: is there an association? Pediatrics 2009;123(2):e228–34.
17. Scott RM, Smith ER. Moyamoya disease and moyamoya syndrome. N Engl J Med 2009;360(12):1226–37.

18. Scott RM, Smith JL, Robertson RL, et al. Long-term outcome in children with moyamoya syndrome after cranial revascularization by pial synangiosis. J Neurosurg 2004;100(2 Suppl Pediatrics):142–9.

19. Rafay MF, Armstrong D, deVeber G, et al. Craniocervical arterial dissection in children: clinical and radiographic presentation and outcome. J Child Neurol 2006;21(1):8–16.

20. Fullerton HJ, Johnston SC, Smith WS. Arterial dissection and stroke in children. Neurology 2001;57(7):1155–60.

21. Hoppe C. Defining stroke risk in children with sickle cell anaemia. Br J Haematol 2004;128(6):751–66.

22. Ohene-Frempong K, Weiner SK, Sleeper LA, et al. Cerebrovascular accidents in sickle cell disease: rates and risk factors. Blood 1998;91(1):288–94.

23. Leikin SL, Gallagher D, Kinney TR, et al. Mortality in children and adolescents with sickle cell disease. Cooperative Study of Sickle Cell Disease. Pediatrics 1989;84:500–8.

24. Adams RJ, McKie VC, Nichols F, et al. The use of transcranial ultrasonography to predict stroke in sickle cell disease. N Engl J Med 1992;326(9):605–10.

25. National Institute for Health. National Heart, Lung, and Blood Institute (NHLBI). The management of sickle cell disease. 4th edition, 2002. Available at: http://www.nhlbi.nih.gov/health/prof/blood/sickle/sc_mngt.pdf. Accessed February 1, 2012.

26. Adams RJ, McKie VC, Hsu L, et al. Prevention of a first stroke by transfusions in children with sickle cell anemia and abnormal results on transcranial Doppler ultrasonography. N Engl J Med 1998;339(1):5–11.

27. Adams RJ, Brambilla D, Optimizing Primary Stroke Prevention in Sickle Cell Anemia (STOP 2) Trial Investigators. Discontinuing prophylactic transfusions used to prevent stoke in sickle cell disease. N Engl J Med 2005;353(26): 2769–78.

28. National Heart, Lung, and Blood Institute (NHLBI) press release, 6/4/2010. Available at: http://public.nhlbi.nih.gov/newsroom/home/GetPressRelease.aspx?id=2709. Accessed February 1, 2012.

29. Domi T, Edgell DS, McCrindle BW, et al. Frequency, predictors, and neurologic outcomes of vaso-occlusive strokes associated with cardiac surgery in children. Pediatrics 2008;122(6):1292–8.

30. Chan AK, deVeber G. Prothrombotic disorders and ischemic stroke in children. Semin Pediatr Neurol 2000;7(4):301–8.

31. Barnes C, Deveber G. Prothrombotic abnormalities in childhood ischaemic stroke. Thromb Res 2006;118(1):67–74.

32. Kenet G, Lütkhoff LK, Albisetti M, et al. Impact of thrombophilia on risk of arterial ischemic stroke or cerebral sinovenous thrombosis in neonates and children: a systematic review and meta-analysis of observational studies. Circulation 2010;121(16):1838–47.

33. Maguire JL, deVeber G, Parkin PC. Association between iron-deficiency anemia and stroke in young children. Pediatrics 2007;120(5):1053–7.

34. Hartfield DS, Lowry NJ, Keene DL, et al. Iron deficiency: a cause of stroke in infants and children. Pediatr Neurol 1997;16(1):50–3.

35. Munot P, De Vile C, Hemingway C, et al. Severe iron deficiency anaemia and ischaemic stroke in children. Arch Dis Child 2011;96(3):276–9.

36. Monagle P, Chalmers E, Chan A, et al. Antithrombotic therapy in neonates and children: American College of Chest Physicians evidence-based clinical practice guidelines (8th edition). Chest 2008;133(Suppl 6):887S–968S.

37. Bernard TJ, Goldenberg NA, Tripputi M, et al. Anticoagulation in childhood-onset arterial ischemic stroke with non-moyamoya arteriopathy: findings from the Colorado and German (COAG) collaboration. Stroke 2009;40(8):2869–71.

38. Ganesan V, Prengler M, Wade A, et al. Clinical and radiological recurrence after childhood arterial ischemic stroke. Circulation 2006;114(20):2170–7.

39. Strater R, Kurnik K, Heller C, et al. Aspirin versus low-dose low-molecular-weight heparin: antithrombotic therapy in pediatric ischemic stroke patients: a prospective follow-up study. Stroke 2001;32(11):2554–8.

40. Amlie-Lefond C, deVeber G, Chan AK, et al. Use of alteplase in childhood arterial ischaemic stroke: a multicentre, observational, cohort study. Lancet Neurol 2009; 8(6):530–6.

41. Janjua N, Nasar A, Lynch JK, et al. Thrombolysis for ischemic stroke in children: data from the nationwide inpatient sample. Stroke 2007;38(6):1850–4.

42. Amlie-Lefond C, Chan AK, Kirton A, et al. Thrombolysis in acute childhood stroke: design and challenges of the thrombolysis in pediatric stroke clinical trial. Neuroepidemiology 2009;32(4):279–86.

43. Intracerebral hemorrhage after intravenous t-PA therapy for ischemic stroke. The NINDS t-PA Stroke Study Group. Stroke 1997;28(11):2109–18.

44. Kuhle S, Mitchell L, Andrew M, et al. Urgent clinical challenges in children with ischemic stroke: analysis of 1065 patients from the 1–800-NOCLOTS pediatric stroke telephone consultation service. Stroke 2006;37(1):116–22.

45. Ronning OM, Guldvog B. Should stroke victims routinely receive supplemental oxygen? A quasi-randomized controlled trial. Stroke 1999;30(10):2033–7.

46. Badjatia N. Hyperthermia and fever control in brain injury. Crit Care Med 2009; 37(Suppl 7):S250–7.

47. Schwab S, Georgiadis D, Berrouschot J, et al. Feasibility and safety of moderate hypothermia after massive hemispheric infarction. Stroke 2001; 32(9):2033–5.

48. Chalmers EA. Perinatal stroke-risk factors and management. Br J Haematol 2005; 130(3):333–43.

49. Chabrier S, Husson B, Dinomais M, et al. New insights (and new interrogations) in perinatal arterial ischemic stroke. Thromb Res 2011;127(1):13–22.

50. Rutherford MA, Ramenghi LA, Cowan FM, et al. Neonatal stroke. Arch Dis Child Fetal Neonatal Ed. Published online August 17, 2011.

51. Beslow LA, Smith SE, Vossough A, et al. Hemorrhagic transformation of childhood arterial ischemic stroke. Stroke 2011;42(4):941–6.

52. deVeber G, Andrew M, Adams C, et al. Cerebral sinovenous thrombosis in children. N Engl J Med 2001;345(6):417–23.

53. Dlamini N, Billinghurst L, Kirkham FJ. Cerebral venous sinus (sinovenous) thrombosis in children. Neurosurg Clin N Am 2010;21(3):511–27.

54. Saposnik G, Barinagarrementeria F, Brown RD Jr, et al. Diagnosis and management of cerebral venous thrombosis: a statement for healthcare professionals from the American Heart Association/American Stroke Association. Stroke 2011;42(4):1158–92.

55. Moharir MD, Shroff M, Stephens D, et al. Anticoagulants in pediatric cerebral sinovenous thrombosis: a safety and outcome study. Ann Neurol 2010;67(5):590–9.

56. Kersbergen KJ, de Vries LS, van Straaten HL, et al. Anticoagulation therapy and imaging in neonates with a unilateral thalamic hemorrhage due to cerebral sinovenous thrombosis. Stroke 2009;40(8):2754–60.

57. Lo WD. Childhood hemorrhagic stroke: an important but understudied problem. J Child Neurol 2011;26(9):1174–85.

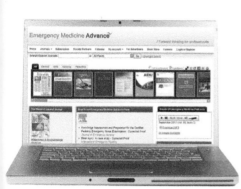

Printed and bound by CPI Group (UK) Ltd, Croydon, CR0 4YY

03/10/2024

01040459-0007

Box 6
Emergent neuroimaging for suspected pediatric stroke

CT brain without contrast to exclude hemorrhage and mass effect if MRI is unattainable

- Consider CT angiography/venography

MRI with diffusion-weighted sequences

- Excludes hemorrhage
- Defines the extent and territory of infarct
- Diffusion imaging differentiates acute from chronic infarct

MR angiography (MRA)

- Defines vascular anatomy of the circle of Willis vessels and neck vessels

MR venography (MRV)

- Excludes CVST

Axial T1-weighted MRI of the neck with fat saturation sequence

- Excludes CCAD

Conventional angiography

- Consider if normal coagulation and no obvious cause for hemorrhage on MRA and MRV or ischemic stroke with normal MRA, MRV, and T1 MRI with fat saturation of neck

Data from Pappachan J, Kirkham FJ. Cerebrovascular disease and stroke. Arch Dis Child 2008;93(10):890.

In addition, MR angiography (MRA) of the head is used to evaluate the intracranial large arteries, whereas MRA of the neck helps evaluate the extracranial large arteries. Axial T1-weighted MRI of the neck with fat saturation should be performed to exclude arterial dissection. MR venography (MRV) should be considered to look for CVST. MRA or conventional angiography (CA) is rarely used in neonates; however, MRA and MRV will provide the best means to evaluate for vascular trauma and congenital vascular anomalies causing perinatal stroke.[62]

Typical MRI sequences require 3 to 5 minutes each to acquire, and the assessment for cerebrovascular disease takes from 15 to 35 minutes. Patient movement during image acquisition will render most sequences useless. Consequently, successful MRI requires considerable patient cooperation, and most children require sedation.[1]

In contrast, CT scans can be completed in a matter of seconds, often reducing the need for sedation. CT uses ionizing radiation, a particular concern for children because recent studies have demonstrated a relative increased lifetime cancer risk even with low radiation doses. Unenhanced CT is a sensitive means of detecting intracranial hemorrhage and mass effect. However in the early acute phase, AIS is often missed until at least 6 hours after onset of symptoms.[1] Although CVST is sometimes evident on unenhanced CT, these lesions are more reliably identified with MRI and MRV by demonstrating a lack of flow in the cerebral veins with or without brain infarction. Unenhanced CT scans may detect deep venous thrombosis as linear densities in the deep or cortical veins. As the thrombus becomes less dense, contrast may demonstrate the empty delta sign, a filling defect, in the posterior part of the sagittal sinus. CT scan with contrast misses the diagnosis of CVST in up to 40% of patients.[53]

CT is the ideal imaging technique in unstable patients or patients in whom acute intracranial hemorrhage is likely. Children who have cochlear implants, cardiac